Keto Diet:

100+ Low-Carb Healthy Ketogenic Recipes & Desserts That Can Change Your Life! (Keto Cookbook, Lose Weight, Burn Fat, Fight Disease, Ketogenic Fat Bombs)

Kevin Gise © 2017

Disclaimer:

This book is for informational purposes only and the author, his agents, heirs, and assignees do not accept any responsibilities for any liabilities, actual or alleged, resulting from the use of this information.

This report is not "professional advice." The author encourages the reader to seek advice from a professional where any reasonably prudent person would do so. While every reasonable attempt has been made to verify the information contained in this eBook, the author and his affiliates cannot assume any responsibility for errors, inaccuracies or omissions, including omissions in transmission or reproduction.

Any references to people, events, organizations, or business entities are for educational and illustrative purposes only, and no intent to falsely characterize, recommend, disparage, or injure is intended or should be so construed. Any results stated or implied are consistent with general results, but this means results can and will vary. The author, his agents, and assigns, make no promises or guarantees, stated or implied. Individual results will vary and this work is supplied strictly on an "at your own risk" basis.

Introduction

First off, thanks for purchasing my book "Keto Diet: 100+ Low-Carb Healthy Ketogenic Recipes & Desserts That Can Change Your Life!" By picking up this recipe book it show that you're willing and ready to make a change in your diet and start living a more health conscious lifestyle. My goal is for you to use the recipes I've included to improve your eating habits and change your life for the better. I hope that you get as much out of the ketogenic diet as I have over the years. This diet helped me to drop a significant amount of weight and improve my blood pressure and blood sugar levels in the process. Today, I'm filled with more energy than ever before and I'm able to lead the life I've always wanted because of all the health benefits following this diet provided.

I hope you like all the recipes I've included. There's so many great meal options you can prepare for you and your family on the keto diet. These recipes should helped get you started off on the right foot.

I'm excited to begin. Let's get to it!

Chapter One: Keto Diet Breakfast Recipes

In this section, I will show you 30+ ketogenic breakfast recipes you can cook for yourself. I'll include a few basic recipes and a few more advanced recipes. That way no matter what your level in the kitchen you'll be able to prepare a healthy low-carb high-fat keto meal to keep you on track with your diet.

Morning Detox Tea (Serves 1)

Ingredients:

1 cup of Warm Water

2 tablespoons of Apple Cider Vinegar

1 tablespoon of Honey

2 tablespoons of Lemon Juice

1 dash of Cayenne

1 teaspoon of Cinnamon

Directions:

1. Combine all your ingredients and stir well.

2. Serve!

Keto Egg Porridge (Serves 1)

Ingredients:

2 Organic Free-Range Eggs

1/3 cup of Organic Heavy Cream Without Food Additives

2 tablespoons of Grass-Fed Butter

2 packages of NuStevia

Ground Organic Ceylon Cinnamon

Directions:

1. Combine your eggs, cream, and the sweetener in your small-sized bowl. Give your mixture a little whisk.

2. Melt your butter in a medium-sized saucepan over a medium-high heat. Don't let the butter get any brown color, but just melt. Turn your heat to the minimum once your butter is melted.

3. Add your egg and cream mixture. Cook, all the time mixing along the bottom until your mixture thickens and starts curdling.

4. When you see the first signs of curdling, i.e. those tiny grains, take your saucepan immediately off the heat.

5. Transfer your porridge to a serving bowl. Sprinkle cinnamon on top.

6. Serve!

Keto Waffles (Serves 5)

Ingredients:

5 Eggs (Separated)

5 tablespoons of Granulated Sweetener

4 tablespoons of Coconut Flour

2 teaspoons of Vanilla

3 tablespoons of Full Fat Milk or Cream

1 teaspoon of Baking Powder

4 1/2 ounces of Melted Butter

Directions:

1. In your first bowl, whisk your egg whites until firm and form stiff peaks.

2. In your second bowl, mix your egg yolks, sweetener, coconut flour, and baking powder.

3. Add your melted butter slowly, mixing to ensure it is a smooth consistency.

4. Add your milk and vanilla, mix together well.

5. Gently fold spoons of your whisked egg whites into your yolk mixture. Try to keep as much of the air and fluffiness as possible.

6. Place enough of your waffle mixture into the warm waffle maker to make one waffle. Cook until golden.

7. Repeat until all your mixture has been used.

8. Serve!

Keto Pumpkin Spiced Granola (Serves 8)

Ingredients:

Dry Ingredients:

1 cup of Whole Almonds

1/2 cup of Pecan Nuts

1/2 cup of Macadamia Nuts

1 cup of Flaked Dried Coconut (Unsweetened)

1 cup of Shredded Dried Coconut (Unsweetened)

1/4 cup of Chia Seeds (Whole or Ground)

1/2 cup of Pumpkin Seeds

1/2 cup of Vanilla or Plain Whey Protein

1 tablespoon + 1 teaspoon of Pumpkin Pie Spice Mix

1/4 cup of Erythritol or Swerve

1/4 teaspoon of Salt

1 Large Egg White

1/2 cup of Pumpkin Puree

1/4 cup of Melted Extra-Virgin Coconut Oil

15 drops of Liquid Stevia Extract

Directions:

1. Preheat your oven to 300 degrees. Roughly chop your almonds, macadamia nuts, and pecans and place them in your mixing bowl.

2. Add your shredded and flaked coconut, pumpkin seeds, chia seeds, protein powder, and Erythritol.

3. Add your pumpkin spice mix and salt. Pour in your egg white, melted coconut oil, and add stevia. Mix until well combined.

4. Add your pumpkin puree and mix well.

5. Place your granola mixture on your baking tray and spread evenly over the surface. Place in your oven and bake for approximately 30 to 40 minutes or until crispy.

6. Once done, remove from your oven and set to the side on your cooling rack. Once chilled, transfer into your jar or airtight container and keep at room temperature for up to a month.

7. On the side add your cream, almond milk, yogurt, or coconut milk.

8. Serve!

Fisherman's Eggs (Serves 1)

Ingredients:

2 Organic Cage Free Eggs

1/2 cup of Organic Arugula

56 grams of Sardines In Olive Oil

2 1/2 tablespoons of Marinated Artichoke Hearts

Pinch of Celtic Sea Salt

Fresh Black Pepper

Directions:

1. Preheat your oven to 375 degrees.

2. Put your sardines in the bottom of your small-sized oven proof stoneware.

3. Break your eggs on top of your sardines.

4. Add your arugula and the artichokes on top.

5. Sprinkle with your salt and pepper.

6. Bake at 375 degrees for about 10 minutes or until your eggs reach desired doneness.

7. Serve!

Coconut Blueberry Porridge (Serves 2)

Ingredients:

Porridge:

1/4 cup of Coconut Flour

1/4 cup of Ground Flaxseed

1 teaspoon of Vanilla Extract

1 cup of Almond Milk

10 drops of Liquid Stevia

1 teaspoon of Cinnamon

Pinch of Salt

Toppings:

2 ounces of Blueberries

2 tablespoons of Butter

1 ounce of Shaved Coconut

2 tablespoons of Pumpkin Seeds

Directions:

1. Place a cup of your almond milk over a low heat.

2. Add in your flaxseed, salt, cinnamon, and coconut flour. Whisk to break any clumps.

3. Heat until bubbling slightly. Add your vanilla extract and liquid Stevia.

4. When your mixture is thick turn off your flame and add in your toppings.

5. Serve!

Steak & Eggs (Serves 1)

Ingredients:

3 Eggs

1 tablespoon of Butter

1/4 Avocado

4 ounces of Sirloin

Salt

Pepper

Directions:

1. Melt your butter in your pan. Fry your eggs until whites have been set and the yolk is done to your desired preference. Season them with your pepper and salt.

2. Cook your sirloin in another pan until desired preference. Slice into small-sized strips and season with your pepper and salt.

3. Slice up your avocado and add to your dish.

4. Serve!

Fried Crusty Cheddar (Serves 1)

Ingredients:

1 Egg

2 slices of Cheddar Cheese

1 teaspoon of Almond Flour

1 teaspoon of Ground Flaxseed

1 tablespoon of Olive Oil

1 teaspoon of Hemp Nuts

Salt

Pepper

Directions:

1. Heat your olive oil in your frying pan over a medium heat.

2. Whisk your egg with your pepper and salt.

3. Mix your flaxseed with hemp nuts and almond flour.

4. Coat your cheddar slices with your egg mixture and then with your dry mixture.

5. Fry them for approximately 3 minutes on both sides.

6. Serve!

Ricotta Cheese w/ Vanilla (Serves 1)

Ingredients:

7 ounces of 2% Fat Ricotta Cheese

1 tablespoon of Creme Fraiche

1 sachet of Vanilla Flavoring

Directions:

1. Mix your ricotta with your creme fraiche and vanilla flavoring.

2. Serve!

Crunchy Keto Cereal w/ Strawberries

Ingredients:

1 package of Bob's Red Mill Flaked Coconut

2 Medium Strawberries

Ground Cinnamon

Unsweetened Almond Milk

Stevia

Parchment Paper or Coconut Oil

Directions:

1. Preheat your oven to 350 degrees.

2. Line your cookie sheet with parchment paper. If no parchment paper grease your cooking sheet using your coconut oil.

3. Pour your coconut flakes on your cookie sheet.

4. Cook in your oven for approximately 5 minutes.

5. Shuffle your flakes around and continue cooking until they are a lightly toasted and lightly tan.

6. Take your flakes out of your oven.

7. Sprinkle them lightly with cinnamon. Can also sprinkle lightly with Stevia.

8. Throw your toasted chips in your bowl and pour your almond milk over them.

9. Slice up 2 strawberries as the garnish on top.

10. Serve!

Keto French Toast (Serves 4)

Ingredients:

8 Large Eggs

2 teaspoon of Baking Powder

3/4 cup of Unsweetened Almond Milk

1/4 cup of Coconut Flour

1 tablespoon of Swerve or Sugar Equivalent

1/4 cup of Melted Butter

1 teaspoon of Vanilla Extract

1/4 cup of Fresh Whole Butter

1/2 cup of Heavy Whipping Cream

2 grams of Salt

Directions:

1. Mix your coconut flour, baking powder, salt, and sugar.

2. In a different bowl, whisk together 4 of your 8 eggs. Add 1/4 cup of your almond milk and vanilla. Whisk together.

3. Add your dry and wet ingredients together and whisk. Continue to do so while pouring in your melted butter.

4. Grease your 12 microwave safe containers. Use wide containers.

5. Microwave your muffins. For each additional muffin add a minute to microwave time. I made 2 batches of 6 muffins with 6 minutes for each batch.

6. While your muffins are cooking, in your large-sized mixing bowl, whisk together your other 4 eggs, 1/2 cup of heavy cream, and 1/2 cup of almond milk.

7. As muffins come out of your microwave, pop them out of your containers and allow them to cool for a minute. When they are cool enough, add to your egg mixture and allow them to sit for a couple of minutes. Flip them occasionally while letting them sit.

8. Once they've absorbed some of the mixture, heat up your large-sized skillet over a medium-low heat. Add some fresh butter and melt it.

9. Fry your muffins like you would French toast.

10. Serve!

Clouds of Eggs (Serves 4)

Ingredients:

4 Large Eggs

2 tablespoons of Parmesan Cheese

2 slices of Bacon

Salt

Pepper

Garlic Powder

Onion Powder

Directions:

1. Split your egg yolks from your egg whites.

2. Cut up your bacon and cook for some bacon bits.

3. Put your eggs in your bowl and then whip them until they are stiff.

4. Shred your Parmesan cheese into your egg whites and then add in your bacon bits.

5. Split your egg white into 4 separate mounds on parchment paper or a silicon mat.

6. Bake your egg whites for approximately 5 minutes at approximately 350 degrees until they are set.

7. Put egg yolk into each of your mounds.

8. Bake your egg whites until brown.

9. Serve!

Breakfast Peanut Butter Bars (Serves 12)

Ingredients:

2 Egg Whites

1/2 cup of Flaxseed Meal

1 cup of Chunky Peanut Butter

1/2 cup of Sweetener

1/2 cup of Sugar-Free Chocolate Chips

1/2 cup of Almond Meal

1/2 cup of Almonds

1/2 teaspoon of Chia Seeds

1/2 cup of Cashews

Directions:

1. Preheat your oven to 350 degrees. Line your 8x8-inch pan or dish with parchment paper.

2. In your large-sized bowl mix together all your ingredients until they are well combined.

3. Pour your mixture into your pan and press your mixture into the pan so that it's flat.

4. Bake for approximately 10 to 15 minutes.

5. Allow it to cool down and refrigerate for approximately 30 minutes.

6. Cut into 12 equal size bars.

7. Keep your bars refrigerated.

8. Serve!

Strawberry Almond Milk (Serves 2)

Ingredients:

4 ounces of Heavy Cream

16 ounces of Unsweetened Almond Milk

1/4 cup of Unsweetened Frozen Strawberries

1 scoop of Whey Vanilla Isolate Powder

Stevia or Low-Carb Sweetener

Directions:

1. Put each of your ingredients in your blender.

2. Blend until your mixture is smooth.

3. Serve!

Snickerdoodle Crepes (Serves 8)

Ingredients:

Crepes:

6 Eggs

1 teaspoon of Cinnamon

5 ounces of Softened Cream Cheese

1 tablespoon of Sugar Substitute

Butter

Filling:

8 tablespoons of Softened Butter

1/3 cup of Granulated Sugar Substitute

1 tablespoon of Cinnamon

Directions:

1. Blend all your crepe ingredients together except for your butter. Place them in your blender or your magic bullet until they are smooth. Allow your batter to rest for approximately 5 minutes.

2. Heat your butter in your non-stick pan over a medium heat until it is sizzling. Pour in enough batter to form a 6-inch crepe. Proceed to cook for approximately 2 minutes before flipping and cooking the other side for an additional minute. Remove your crepe and place on your warm plate. This should make about 8 crepes.

3. In your small-sized bowl, mix together your cinnamon and sweetener until they are combined. Stir half of your mixture into the softened butter until it is smooth.

4. Spread a tablespoon of your butter mixture in the middle of your crepe. Roll it up and sprinkle an additional teaspoon of mixture onto it.

5. Serve!

Breakfast Chia Bowl (Serves 2)

Ingredients:

2 tablespoons of Pure Maple Syrup

2 cups of Unsweetened NonDairy Milk

1 teaspoon of Vanilla Extract

1/4 cup of Whole Chia Seeds

Toppings:

Fresh Fruit

Cinnamon (Optional)

Nuts (Optional)

Directions:

1. Combine your milk, seeds, vanilla, and syrup in your bowl and stir it all together.

2. Allow it to stand for approximately 30 minutes. Whisk together to keep your seeds from getting clumped together. Move to an air tight container. Cover and refrigerate overnight.

3. Divide between 2 different bowls and add your choice of toppings.

4. Serve!

Spicy Shrimp Omelet (Serves 2)

Ingredients:

10 Large Shrimp

6 Eggs

1/4 Onion

4 Grape Tomatoes

1 teaspoon of Cayenne

1 tablespoon of Sriracha Salt

Sprig of Parsley

Handful of Spinach

Directions:

1. Chop your onion and slice your grape tomatoes lengthwise in half.

2. Fire your pan to a medium heat. Add your onions and salt. Add your grape tomatoes cut side down so they can roast a little bit.

3. When your onions get translucent add in your spinach and allow it to shrink and wilt enough for some of your shrimp to fit in.

4. Throw your shrimp in.

5. Crack each egg leaving room for all of them. Take your spoon and jiggle around the whites so they grab everything that is underneath them.

6. Place a lid on your pan. Allow your omelet to cook for approximately 6 to 8 minutes. Watch your eggs, once thin film of white has covered the yolks they're ready. If eggs are still runny let them cook a bit longer.

7. Once your omelet is done, run your knife across each of the yolks and allow them to ooze out onto your whole omelet. Garnish with your parsley.

8. Serve!

Orange Cooler Creamsicle (Serves 2)

Ingredients:

1/4 cup of Unsweetened Frozen Blueberries

16 ounces of Unsweetened Almond Milk

1 scoop of Whey Dreamsicle Powder

4 ounces of Heavy Cream

Stevia or Low-Carb Sweetener

1/2 cup of Crushed Ice

Directions:

1. Put each of your ingredients in your blender.

2. Blend until your mixture is smooth.

3. Serve!

Almond Bacon Waffles (Serves 2)

Ingredients:

2 Eggs

3/4 cup of Almond Flour

4 slices of Bacon

1 1/2 teaspoons of Splenda

1 1/2 teaspoons of Baking Soda

5 tablespoons of Melted Unsalted Butter

Directions:

1. Cook your bacon until it's crisp.

2. Place your eggs in your warm water to get them heated up.

3. Mix your dry ingredients. This includes your Splenda, baking powder, and almond flour.

4. Add your 2 eggs and mix together well.

5. Microwave your butter and add it to your mix.

6. Preheat your waffle maker.

7. Once your waffle maker is heated, spray with your Pam and fill with your batter. Add in your bacon.

8. Cook your waffle following your waffle maker's instructions. Many will vary on time and temperature.

9. Remove your waffle and add any desired toppings.

10. Serve!

Keto Pumpkin Bread Loaf (Serves 10)

Ingredients:

3 Large Egg Whites

1/2 cup of Pumpkin Puree

1 1/2 cups of Almond Flour

1/2 cup of Coconut Milk

1/4 cup of Swerve Sweetener

2 teaspoons of Baking Powder

1/4 cup of Psyllium Husk Powder

1 1/2 teaspoons of Pumpkin Pie Spice

1/2 teaspoon of Kosher Salt

Directions:

1. Measure your dry ingredients into your sifter.

2. Sift your ingredients into your large-sized bowl.

3. Preheat your oven to 350 degrees. Fill your 9x9-inch baking dish with a cup of water and put on the bottom rack of your oven.

4. Add your coconut milk to your bowl and mix together.

5. Whip your egg whites in a different bowl.

6. Fold in 1/3 of your eggs whites to your dough mixture so the moisture gets absorbed. Add the rest of your egg whites and fold them gently into your dough.

7. Grease your bread loaf pan with coconut oil or butter. Spread out your dough into your bread pan.

8. Bake for approximately 75 minutes.

9. Remove from your oven and allow it to cool.

10. Slice into 10 equal pieces.

11. Serve!

Cream, Flaxseed, & Goji Cup (Serves 1)

Ingredients:

1 teaspoon of Dark Unsweetened Cocoa Powder

1 ounce of Ground Flaxseed

100 milliliters of 35% Fat Cooking Cream

1 tablespoon of Goji Berries

Freshly Brewed Coffee

Liquid Sweetener

Directions:

1. Mix your ground flaxseed, cream, and cocoa until your flaxseed is covered. Add your liquid sweetener for more sweetness.

2. Add your coffee. If you don't like coffee add a couple spoons worth of water.

3. Add your Goji berries.

4. Serve!

Heavenly Chocolate Milk (Serves 2)

Ingredients:

16 ounces of Unsweetened Almond Milk

4 ounces of Heavy Cream

1 scoop of Whey Chocolate Isolate Powder

Stevia or Low-Carb Sweetener

1/2 cup of Crushed Ice (Optional)

Directions:

1. Put each of your ingredients in your blender.

2. Blend until it is smooth.

3. Serve!

Lemon Blueberry Muffins (Serves 15)

Ingredients:

2 Eggs

1/8 cup of Melted Butter

2 cups of Almond Flour

4 ounces of Fresh Blueberries

1 cup of Heavy Cream

1/2 teaspoon of Baking Soda

1/2 teaspoon of Lemon Flavoring or Extract

5 packets of Stevia or Splenda

1/2 teaspoon of Dried Lemon Zest

1/4 teaspoon of Salt

Directions:

1. Preheat your oven 350 degrees. Place some cupcake paper in each muffin hole of a normal sized 12 serving muffin pan. This recipe will make 15 muffins so you'll need two pans.

2. Mix your cream and almond flour.

3. Add in your eggs one by one. Stir until they are all mixed.

4. Add your sweetener, butter, spices, flavoring, and baking soda. Mix together.

5. Add your blueberries. Stir until they are all distributed evenly.

6. Spoon your mixture into your pans. Fill each spot until it is 1/2 full.

7. Bake for around 20 minutes. Should be golden colored when finished.

8. Take out of your oven and allow it to cool off.

9. Serve!

Low-Carb Blueberry Muffins (Serves 6)

Ingredients:

3 Large Organic Eggs

5 tablespoons of Organic Coconut Flour

1/4 cup of Heavy Cream

1/2 cup of Frozen Organic Blueberries

1/3 cup of Erythritol Crystals

Directions:

1. Preheat your oven to 350 degrees.

2. Line your muffin pan with some paper liners.

3. In your large-sized bowl, add your eggs, erythritol, and cream. Whisk together until it is mixed well.

4. Add your coconut flour to your egg mix and whisk until it is smooth.

5. Allow it to rest for 5 minutes until your batter thickens. Add your frozen blueberries and mix in well.

6. Scoop your batter into your muffin cups.

7. Bake for approximately 25 to 30 minutes.

8. Allow it to cool.

9. Serve!

Cinnamon Instant Oatmeal

Ingredients:

2/3 cup of Golden Flax Meal

2/3 cup of Chia Seeds

2 tablespoons of Unsweetened Coconut Milk

2/3 cup of Unsweetened Coconut

1/2 cup of Hot Water

2 tablespoons of Ground Cinnamon

Sweetener

Directions:

1. Combine your golden flax meal, chia seed, cinnamon, and unsweetened coconut in an airtight container.

2. Scoop out your 1/2 cup of this mixture and keep the rest stored in your container.

3. Pour 1/2 cup of water on your mixture and allow it to sit between 3 and 5 minutes.

4. Add your sweetener and coconut milk into your bowl. Stir to combine.

5. Serve!

Perfected Scrambled Eggs (Serves 2)

Ingredients:

6 Eggs

2 tablespoons of Butter

4 strips of Bacon

2 tablespoons of Sour Cream

1/2 teaspoon of Garlic Powder

1/2 teaspoon of Onion Powder

1/4 teaspoon of Paprika

1/2 teaspoon of Salt

1/4 teaspoon of Black Pepper

Directions:

1. Crack your eggs into an ungreased, cold pan and then add your butter. Wait to mix your eggs until you put the heat on. Don't season your eggs until after you cooked them. It will break the eggs down and make them watery instead of creamy.

2. Put your pan on a medium-high heat. Start stirring your butter and eggs together using preferably a silicone spatula. While stirring your eggs, cook some bacon strips in a different pan to your desired level of crispiness.

3. Alternate stirring your eggs both on heat and off the heat. A few seconds on and a few seconds off the flame. If your eggs begin cooking in a thin, dry looking layer at the bottom of your pan, take if off heat. Scrape it using your spatula and that thin layer should regain some of its creaminess.

4. Once the eggs are almost done turn off the flame. Your eggs will cook a little more due to residual heat in your pan.

5. Add 2 tablespoons of your sour cream. Season your eggs using the pepper, salt, paprika, onion powder, and garlic powder.

6. You can add in a couple stalks of chopped green onion for some contrasting flavor.

7. Serve!

Blueberry Almond Milk (Serves 2)

Ingredients:

1/4 cup of Unsweetened Frozen Blueberries

4 ounces of Heavy Cream

16 ounces of Unsweetened Almond Milk

1 scoop of Whey Vanilla Isolate Powder

Stevia or Low-Carb Sweetener

Directions:

1. Put each of your ingredients in your blender.

2. Blend until your mixture is smooth.

3. Serve!

Gluten Free Banana Bread (Serves 8)

Ingredients:

Wet Ingredients:

3 Ripe Bananas

1/4 teaspoon of Vanilla Extract

1/4 cup of Honey

2 tablespoons of Coconut Oil

1 Juiced Orange

Pinch of Orange Zest

Dry Ingredients:

1/2 teaspoon of Baking Soda

1 1/3 cup of Almond Flour

3/4 teaspoon of Cinnamon

1 teaspoon of Xanthan Gum

1/8 teaspoon of Cayenne

1 teaspoon of Baking Powder

1/2 teaspoon of Salt

Fold-Ins:

2 Grated Carrots

3/ cup of Flaxseeds

3/4 cup of Chopped Walnuts

1/4 teaspoon of Grated Fresh Ginger

Topping:

Honey

Coconut Butter

Directions:

1. Preheat your oven to 410 degrees.

2. Mash your bananas until they are in a thick wet mush.

3. Take your zest from the peel of your orange. Cut in half and juice the whole thing into your bananas.

4. Add your vanilla extract, honey, and coconut oil.

5. Add in all your dry ingredients.

6. Shred your ginger carrots to fold in. Chop your walnuts and throw them into your mixture.

7. Fold in the rest of your ingredients.

8. Grease your medium 8x4-inch bread pan with butter or coconut oil. Pour in your batter.

9. Bake for approximately 25 minutes at 410 degrees. Lower to 350 degrees and bake for another 30 minutes.

10. Allow your bread to cool. Drizzle your honey on top. Slice into 8 pieces.

11. Serve!

Bacon Hash (Serves 2)

Ingredients:

4 Eggs

6 slices of Bacon

1 Small Pepper

1 Small Onion

Jalapeno Slices

Directions:

1. Slice your onion and pepper into a thin strip.

2. Dice your jalapeno slices up as small as you can.

3. Fry all your vegetables in your cast iron pan.

4. Remove when your vegetables are browning and translucent.

5. Chop your bacon using a food processor until it's broken in chunks. Don't overdo it. You don't want it to be a paste.

6. Mix everything together.

7. Cook your hash until your bacon is about to crisp.

8. Fry an egg.

9. Arrange it on your plate and top it with your fried egg.

10. Serve!

High Fiber Coffee & Coconut Cup (Serves 1)

Ingredients:

1 ounce of Ground Flaxseed

1 ounce of Unsweetened Ground Flaxseed

1/2 cup of Unsweetened Black Coffee

1 tablespoon of Coconut Oil

Liquid Sweetener

Directions:

1. Mix your flaxseed and coconut flakes together well.

2. Add your coconut oil. Pour your hot coffee on it and mix. Adjust the level of thickness by adding more still water or coffee.

3. Add 3 to 4 drops of liquid sweetener.

4. Serve!

Iced Matcha Latte (Serves 1)

Ingredients:

1 tablespoon of Coconut Oil

1/8 teaspoon of Vanilla Bean

1 teaspoon of Matcha Powder

1 cup of Unsweetened Cashew Milk

2 Ice Cubes

Directions:

1. Combine all your ingredients in your blender and continue to blend until your ice cubes are broken up.

2. Sprinkle some extra matcha on top as your garnish.

3. Serve!

Chapter Two: Keto Diet Lunch Recipes

In this section, I will show you 20+ ketogenic lunch recipes you can cook for yourself. I'll include a few basic recipes and a few more advanced recipes. That way no matter what your level in the kitchen you'll be able to prepare a healthy low-carb high-fat keto meal to keep you on track with your diet.

Cheddar Broccoli Soup (Serves 4)

Ingredients:

1/2 White Onion

1 cup of Heavy Cream

1 tablespoon of Butter

8 ounces of Cheddar

2 cups of Broth

12 ounces of Broccoli

2 cups of Water

1/4 teaspoon of Xanthan Gum

1/2 teaspoon of Paprika

Salt

Pepper

Directions:

1. Heat your large sized soup pot and add a tablespoon of butter.

2. Saute your garlic and onion until fragrant and your onion looks translucent.

3. Add your broth, cream, and water. Allow it to come to a boil. Season with your salt, paprika, and pepper.

4. While boiling rip your broccoli into florets and measure 12 ounces. Place into boiling soup broth and reduce it to a simmer. Allow your broccoli to cook for approximately 25 minutes.

5. Once your broccoli is cooked, add in 8 ounces of cheddar cheese and stir it in until melted. I prefer cubed cheese but shredded works better as it melts quicker.

6. After your cheese has melted, turn the heat off. Pour the contents into your large-sized blender and continue to blend until the contents are smooth. You can also use an immersion blender if you prefer.

7. When blending, slowly add in a 1/4 teaspoon of your xanthan gum. You should notice your soup thickening.

8. When finished, sprinkle some cheddar cheese on top.

9. Serve!

Caprese Salad (Serves 2)

Ingredients:

1/2 pound of Fresh Mozzarella

1 Large Tomato

1 tablespoon of Olive Oil

1 tablespoon of Balsamic Reduction

4 Basil Leaves

Pinch of Salt

Pinch of Pepper

Directions:

1. Wash then cut your tomato into 1 centimeter sized slices.

2. Do the same thing with your mozzarella.

3. Arrange your ingredients on a plate in an alternating pattern.

4. Add some pepper and salt.

5. Drizzle your olive oil and balsamic reduction on top.

6. Place your basil leaves on top.

7. Serve!

Ham and Cheese Keto Stromboli

Ingredients:

4 ounces of Ham

3 1/2 ounces Cheddar Cheese

4 tablespoons of Almond Flour

1 1/4 cups of Shredded Mozzarella Cheese

1 Large Egg

3 tablespoons of Coconut Flour

1 teaspoon of Italian Seasoning

Pepper

Salt

Directions:

1. Preheat your oven to 400 degrees and in your microwave or toaster oven, melt your mozzarella cheese. Should take about 1 minute in your microwave, and 10-second intervals afterward, or about 10 minutes in an oven, stirring occasionally.

2. Combine your almond and coconut flour, as well as your seasonings in your mixing bowl. I used salt, pepper, and an Italian blend seasoning.

3. When your mozzarella is melted, place that into your flour mixture and begin working it in.

4. After about 1 minute, when your cheese has had a chance to cool down a bit, add in your egg and combine everything together.

5. When everything is combined and you've got a moist dough, transfer it to a flat surface with some parchment paper.

6. Lay your second sheet of parchment paper over your dough ball and use a rolling pin or your hand to flatten it out.

7. Use your pizza cutter or knife to cut diagonal lines beginning from the edges of your dough to the center, leave a row of your dough untouched about 4-inches wide.

8. Alternate laying your ham and cheddar on that uncut stretch of dough.

9. Lift one section of your dough at a time and lay it over the top, covering your filling.

10. Bake it for approximately 15 to 20 minutes until you see it has turned a golden brown color.

11. Serve!

Prosciutto, Caramelized Onion, & Parmesan Braid (Serves 6)

Ingredients:

1 tablespoon of Butter

1 Egg

3 ounces of Prosciutto (Sliced Thinly)

1 Medium Onion (Finely Chopped)

2 cups of Part-Skim Mozzarella Cheese (Finely Grated)

1 tablespoon of Balsamic Vinegar

2 teaspoons of Minced Fresh Basil

1 clove of Crushed Garlic

3/4 cup of Almond Flour

1/2 cup + 1 tablespoon of Finely Grated Parmesan Cheese

1/2 teaspoon of Salt

Freshly Ground Black Pepper

Olive Oil (Optional)

Directions:

1. Preheat your oven to 375 degrees. Have 2 pieces of parchment about 18-inches long, a rolling pin, and a baking sheet set to the side.

2. Heat your large-sized skillet over a medium heat, add your butter. When your butter stops foaming, add your onions. Cook your onions, stirring occasionally until your edges are brown and your onions have caramelized.

3. Add your garlic to your skillet. Cook for 1 minute, stirring constantly. Pour your balsamic vinegar over your onions and cook until almost completely evaporated.

4. Add your prosciutto to your skillet, separating the thin slices as you put them in your skillet. Cook while stirring for about 1 minute. Stir in your basil, then remove your skillet from the heat. Taste and adjust seasoning with salt and pepper. Prosciutto is salty already, so the addition of salt will probably not be necessary.

5. Prepare your double boiler and bring your water in the lower part of your double boiler to a simmer. In the top part of your double boiler, add your mozzarella cheese, the almond flour, and the salt. Stir to evenly distribute.

6. Place the top part of your double boiler containing the almond flour and mozzarella mixture over the bottom part with your simmering water. Heat your mixture, stirring frequently, until your cheese melts and the mixture becomes a dough-like ball. Be careful not to burn yourself with steam escaping from the bottom part of your double boiler.

7. Transfer your mozzarella dough to a piece of parchment paper. Knead it several times to incorporate any stray almond flour into your dough and completely mix your cheese and your almond flour. Pat your dough into an oval shape. Cover your dough with a second piece of parchment and roll out into an oblong shape about 14x9-inches. While rolling your dough out, you may need to straighten the top parchment, then flip the dough over and straighten the bottom parchment. This prevents wrinkles in your dough.

8. Spread your filling along the middle third of the dough, being careful to leave about 1/3 of the dough on both sides. Sprinkle 1/2 cup of your Parmesan cheese over your filling.

9. Cut approximately 1-inch wide strips down the sides going to where your filling starts. Make sure there is an equal number of strips on each side. Crisscross the strips as shown. Before you get to the end, fold the bottom over the filling and cross the last few strips over top.

10. Break your egg into your small-sized bowl. Whisk lightly and brush over your bread. (You will not use the entire egg.) Sprinkle your loaf with your reserved Parmesan cheese and a pinch of freshly ground black pepper on top.

11. Using the parchment the bread is already on, slide your bread onto a baking sheet. Bake in your preheated oven for 18 to 22 minutes or until it is golden brown. Let your bread cool for 5 minutes on the baking sheet, then transfer it to a cutting board using the parchment. Gently remove your parchment from underneath, if desired. Tearing the parchment will make this process easier. On the side add your olive oil for dipping if so desired.

12. Serve!

Avocado Tuna Melt Bites (Serves 12)

Ingredients:

10 ounces of Canned Tuna (Drained)

1/3 cup of Almond Flour

1/4 cup of Mayonnaise

1/4 cup of Parmesan Cheese

1 Medium Avocado (Cubed)

1/2 teaspoon of Garlic Powder

1/2 cup of Coconut Oil

1/4 teaspoon of Onion Powder

Pepper

Salt

Directions:

1. Drain your can of tuna and add it to your large-sized container where you'll be able to mix everything together.

2. Add your mayonnaise, Parmesan cheese, and spices to your tuna and mix together well.

3. Slice your avocado in half, remove the pit, and cube the inside.

4. Add your avocado into your tuna mixture and fold together, trying to not mash your avocado into your mixture.

5. Form your tuna mixture into balls and roll into your almond flour, covering completely. Set to the side.

6. Heat your coconut oil in a pan over a medium heat. Once hot, add your tuna balls and fry until crisp on all sides.

7. Remove from your pan.

8. Serve!

Cheese Stuffed Bacon Wrapped Hot Dogs (Serves 6)

Ingredients:

6 Hot Dogs

2 ounces of Cheddar Cheese

12 slices of Bacon

1/2 teaspoon of Onion Powder

1/2 teaspoon of Garlic Powder

Pepper

Salt

Directions:

1. Preheat your oven to 400 degrees. Make a slit in all of your hot dogs to make room for your cheese.

2. Slice 2 ounces Cheddar cheese from your block into small-sized long rectangles and stuff into your hot dogs.

3. Start by tightly wrapping one slice of your bacon around the hot dog.

4. Continue tightly wrapping the second slice of bacon around your hot dog, slightly overlapping with the first slice.

5. Poke toothpicks through each side of your bacon and hot dog, securing your bacon in place.

6. Set on a wire rack that's on top of your cookie sheet. Season with your garlic powder, onion powder, salt, and pepper.

7. Bake for approximately 35 to 40 minutes, or until your bacon is crispy. Broil your bacon on top if needed.

8. Serve!

Simple Taco Salad (Serves 6)

Ingredients:

32 ounces of Ground Pork

6 teaspoons of McCormick Taco Seasoning

9 ounces of Shredded Cheddar Cheese

6 teaspoons of McCormick Taco Seasoning

12 tablespoons of Salsa

12 tablespoons of Sour Cream

6 Romaine Leafs

Cayenne Pepper

Directions:

1. Brown your pork in your skillet.

2. Add your spices and taco seasoning once your meat is browned.

3. Cook until your taco seasoning is incorporated.

4. Allow it to cool and evenly divide into 6 containers.

5. Add your cheese to each of the containers.

6. Add your Romaine to containers.

7. Add salsa and sour cream to your bowl.

8. Serve!

Easy Tomato Soup (Serves 4)

Ingredients:

1 quart of Tomato Soup

1/4 cup of Olive Oil

4 tablespoons of Butter

2 tablespoons of Apple Cider Vinegar

1/4 cup of Frank's Red Hot Sauce

Spices:

1 teaspoon of Oregano

2 teaspoons of Turmeric

2 teaspoons of Black Pepper

1 tablespoon of Pink Himalayan Sea Salt

Toppings:

4 tablespoons of Creme Fraiche

8 strips of Bacon

Fresh Basil

Green Onion

Directions:

1. Cook your bacon in your pan until it is crisp. Prepare your tomato soup.

2. Combine all your main ingredients in your pot. Set to a medium heat and stir.

3. Add in your spices.

4. Cook until your butter is melted. Don't allow your soup to boil. You want it to get to a nice simmer.

5. Pour into your soup bowls and top with your creme fraiche, green onion, basil, and bacon.

6. Serve!

Low-Carb Chicken Quesadilla (Serves 1)

Ingredients:

2.5 ounces of Grilled Chicken Breast

1/2 Sliced Avocado

1 teaspoon of Chopped Jalapeno

3 ounces of Pepper Jack

1 Low-Carb Wrap

Spices:

1/4 teaspoon of Garlic Powder

1/4 teaspoon of Dried Basil

1/4 teaspoon of Crushed Red Pepper

1/4 teaspoon of Salt

Directions:

1. Grill your chopped chicken breast and spices.

2. Place your wrap on your wide frying pan so it can lie flat. Cook over a medium heat.

3. Cook for approximately 2 minutes and flip your wrap over. Lay out your pepper jack. Leave less than an inch from your edges of the wrap.

4. Add your chopped chicken breast, jalapeno, and sliced avocado to 1/2 of your wrap.

5. Add your cheese.

6. Fold your wrap with your spatula and flatten by pressing down gently. You want your melted cheese to glue it all together.

7. Take out of your pan and cut up into thirds. Feel free to add salsa or sour cream for dipping on the side.

8. Serve!

Spicy Tomato Basil Soup (Serves 6)

Ingredients:

3 pounds of Plum Tomatoes

1 Sweet Onion

6 cloves of Garlic

2 tablespoons of Butter

3 tablespoons of Olive Oil

1/2 cup of Basil

1 quart of Broth

2 tablespoons of Tomato Paste

Spices:

1/2 teaspoon of Thyme

1/2 teaspoon of Paprika

1 tablespoon of Sriracha

1/2 teaspoon of Cayenne

1 teaspoon of Crushed Red Pepper

1/2 teaspoon of Pepper

1 tablespoon of Salt

Directions:

1. Divide your tomatoes into thirds. 1/3 will be saved as fresh tomato and the other 2/3 will be roasted.

2. Wash and dry 8 plum tomatoes. Cut in half lengthwise and lay out on your cookie sheet that has been greased, cut side up. Sprinkle these tomatoes with salt and olive oil and bake them in your oven for approximately 40 minutes at 400 degrees. You'll notice your tomatoes get wrinkled and darker as moisture leaves them.

3. While your tomatoes roast, cut up your sweet onion and squeeze your garlic through your garlic press. Add your tablespoon of olive oil to a big soup pot and cook your garlic and onion until they are translucent and fragrant.

4. Cut your fresh tomatoes into small-sized pieces and throw them into garlic and onion. Pour your broth into the pot and let it come to a boil.

5. Add your basil leaves. Make sure they've been chopped up first. Add some butter and tomato paste to the pot.

6. Add your spices. Make it as hot or spicy as you prefer.

7. Boil your spicy mixture over a medium heat while your tomatoes are roasting.

8. Once tomatoes are finished roasting, take them out and add them into your spicy mixture. Lower the heat to low and allow it to simmer for approximately 40 minutes.

9. Ladle a good portion of your soup into your blender or Nutribullet. Blend for a few seconds. The longer you do this the creamier it will get. Don't blend too long. If using a Nutribullet open your blending cap slowly so the steam is released slowly. If you do it too fast hot soup could shoot out and lead to burns.

10. Top with your green onion, sour cream, or shredded cheese.

11. Serve!

Bacon Wrapped Jalapeno Poppers (Serves 4)

Ingredients:

16 Fresh Jalapenos

16 strips of Bacon

1/4 cup of Shredded Cheddar Cheese

4 ounces of Cream Cheese

1 teaspoon of Paprika

1 teaspoon of Salt

Directions:

1. Preheat your oven to 350 degrees.

2. Slice your pieces of bacon in half.

3. Slice the ends off your jalapenos. Slice each one lengthwise in half. Remove the membranes and seeds with your knife or corer. I suggest wearing gloves to protect your hands.

4. Mix your cheddar cheese and cream cheese together in your bowl.

5. Fill each half of your jalapenos with your cheese mixture.

6. Wrap your jalapenos in bacon.

7. Place your bacon wrapped jalapenos on your baking sheet that is lined with aluminum foil. Leave some room between each jalapeno.

8. Bake for approximately 20 to 25 minutes.

9. Add your paprika, salt, and any other desired spices.

10. Serve!

Low-Carb Keto Pizza (Serves 3)

Ingredients:

Crust:

1 Egg

1 1/4 cup of Shredded Mozzarella

4 tablespoons of Almond Flour

3 tablespoons of Coconut Flour

1/2 teaspoon of Fennel Seed

1 teaspoon of Oregano

1/2 teaspoon of Garlic Powder

1 teaspoon of Crushed Red Pepper

1 teaspoon of Salt

Pizza Toppings:

1/2 cup of Pizza Sauce

6 ounces of Sliced Fresh Mozzarella

3 tablespoons of Ricotta Cheese

2 tablespoons of Sliced Jalapenos

Directions:

Pizza Crust:

1. Preheat your oven to 400 degrees.

2. Melt your shredded cheese in a toaster oven or your microwave until it is malleable and soft.

3. Add your spices.

4. Add your almond flour, eggs, and coconut flour to your melted cheese to combine. Be sure all your ingredients are combined well (heat 10 seconds again if needed).

5. Place your dough between 2 sheets of parchment paper and then roll into your preferred shape. I go with a round shape.

6. Bake at 400 degrees for approximately 12 to 15 minutes or until slightly golden.

Pizza Toppings:

7. Evenly spread out your sauce over your crust. Get sauce as close to your edges as you prefer!

8. Lay out your sliced mozzarella over top your sauce. Add small globs of ricotta all around. You want some in every slice.

9. Add any other desired toppings.

10. Bake your pizza for approximately 10 minutes at 400 degrees until mozzarella is fully melted.

11. Serve!

Spaghetti Squash Lasagna (Serves 12)

Ingredients:

3 pounds of Ground Beef

30 slices of Mozzarella Cheese

2 Large Cooked Spaghetti Squash

40 ounces of Rao's Marinara Sauce

32 ounces of Whole Milk Ricotta Cheese

Directions:

1. Preheat your oven to 375 degrees.

2. Split your spaghetti squash and place them face down in your large-sized glass dish. Fill with water until the meat portion of your squash has been covered.

3. Bake for approximately 45 minutes.

4. While baking begin to brown your meat.

5. Add your meat to your large-sized saucepan. Add your marinara sauce. Set this to the side once hot and mixed together.

6. When your spaghetti squash is finished cooking scrap the meat of your squash from the spaghetti.

7. Assemble your lasagna in your large-sized greased pan. First, start with a layer of spaghetti squash followed by meat sauce, mozzarella, ricotta and repeat from beginning until all your ingredients are used up.

8. Bake for approximately 35 minutes. The top layer of your cheese should have begun to brown.

9. Serve!

Almond Bun Pizza (Serves 4)

Ingredients:

4 ounces of Cheddar

2 Eggs

2 ounces of Jarlsberg

3/4 cup of Almond Meal

5 tablespoons of Butter

1/2 teaspoon of Oregano

1 1/2 teaspoons of Splenda

1/2 teaspoon of Garlic Powder

1 1/2 teaspoons of Baking Powder

1/2 cup of Alfredo Sauce

1/4 teaspoon of Thyme

Directions:

1. Combine your dry ingredients and mix them together well.

2. Be sure your eggs are warmed up placing them in some hot water before using.

3. Add your eggs to your dry ingredients.

4. Melt your butter and add to your mixture.

5. Spray some Pam on your pizza pan and spread your mixture on your pan.

6. Cook for approximately 7 minutes at 350 degrees.

7. Add your Alfredo sauce to your pizza.

8. Add your cheese and any other desired toppings.

9. Broil it for approximately 2 minutes.

10. Serve!

Mushroom & Shrimp Zucchini Pasta (Serves 1)

Ingredients:

12 ounces of Peeled Shrimp

2 tablespoons of Butter

2 tablespoons of Olive Oil

1 Large Zucchini

1/2 pound of White Mushrooms

1/2 cup of Marinara Sauce

Parmesan Cheese

Red Pepper Flakes

Basil

Oregano

Pepper

Salt

Directions:

1. Heat up 2 tablespoons of your olive oil over a medium heat in your large-sized pan. Slice your mushrooms and fry until they've soaked most of your oil up.

2. Add 2 tablespoons of your butter and allow your mushrooms to cook until they turn golden.

3. Add your shrimp and cook for approximately 4 minutes on both sides.

4. While your shrimp are cooking begin making your zoodles using a spiralizer. Twist your zucchini to the spiralizer until it begins to resemble noodles.

5. Once your shrimp have cooked, toss in your zoodles and mix all together. Cook for approximately 2 minutes.

6. Add your marinara sauce and season with red pepper flakes, pepper, salt, oregano, and basil.

7. Toss everything together and sprinkle some Parmesan cheese on top.

8. Serve!

Spaghetti Squash w/ Meatballs (Serves 10)

Ingredients:

Beef Meatballs:

16 ounces of Ground Beef (80/20)

1/3 Onion

1/3 Green Pepper

1 Egg

1 tablespoon of Minced Garlic

2 ounces of Shredded Cheddar Cheese

1 tablespoon of Coconut Flour

Salt

Pepper

Pork Meatballs:

16 ounces of Ground Pork

1 Egg

1/3 Green Pepper

2 ounces of Shredded Monterey Jack Cheese

1/3 Onion

1 tablespoon of Almond Flour

1 tablespoon of Minced Garlic

Salt

Pepper

Chicken Meatballs:

16 ounces of Ground Chicken Thighs

1/3 Green Pepper

1 Egg

1/3 Onion

1 tablespoon of Minced Garlic

2 ounces of Shredded Jarlsberg Cheese

1 tablespoon of Ground Flax Meal

Salt

Pepper

Spaghetti:

2 1/4 pounds of Spaghetti Squash (Cooked and Shredded)

10 teaspoons of Parmesan Cheese

24 ounces of Rao's Homemade Marinara Sauce

Directions:

1. Cut your spaghetti squash in two and scrape out the inside.

2. Place it face down in your glass container. Add some water until it goes above your cut portion.

3. Cook for approximately 45 minutes at 375 degrees.

4. Dice your onions and pepper. Divide up into three separate parts.

5. Combine your beef, 1/3 of your onions and peppers, 1 egg, coconut flour, pepper, salt, garlic, and cheddar cheese.

6. Divide this up into 10 separate meatballs. Should be about 1 1/2 ounces each.

7. Place them on your baking sheet that's been lined with foil.

8. Combine your pork, 1/3 of your onions and peppers, 1 egg, almond flour, pepper, salt, garlic, and Monterey Jack cheese.

9. Divide this up into 10 separate meatballs. Should be about 1 1/2 ounces each.

10. Place them on your baking sheet that's been lined with foil.

11. Combine your pork, 1/3 of your onions and peppers, 1 egg, ground flax meal, pepper, salt, garlic, and Jarlsberg cheese.

12. Divide this up into 10 separate meatballs. Should be about 1 1/2 ounces each.

13. Place them on your baking sheet that's been lined with foil.

14. Cook them at 375 degrees for approximately 25 minutes.

15. Place 1/10 of your spaghetti squash, 1 of each type of meatball, 2 ounces of marinara, and 1 ounce of shredded Parmesan cheese into each container. You'll need 10 containers in total.

16. Serve!

Low-Carb Gnocchi (Serves 2)

Ingredients:

2 cups of Shredded Mozzarella

3 Egg Yolks

1/2 teaspoon of Garlic Powder

1 teaspoon of Salt

Directions:

1. Melt your mozzarella. Separate your egg yolks and beat to combine.

2. Pour 1/2 of your egg yolk mixture into your mozzarella and combine.

3. Once combined, separate it into fourths and then roll each of these fourths into thin long strips. Do this on a piece of parchment paper.

4. Cut 1-inch pieces until you have a lot of cheese gnocchi.

5. Boil your water and drop in gnocchi. Boil them until they start to float. Remove from the heat and drain out your water in your strainer.

6. Fry your gnocchi on each side of your oiled pan until it is cooked.

7. Serve!

Easy Cobb Salad (Serves 1)

Ingredients:

2 ounces of Chicken Breast

1 cup of Spinach

1 Hard Boiled Egg

2 strips of Bacon

1/2 Campari Tomato

1/4 Avocado

1/2 teaspoon of White Vinegar

1 tablespoon of Olive Oil

Directions:

1. Cook your chicken and bacon if not cooked yet.

2. Chop your ingredients up into bite sized pieces.

3. Combine all your ingredients in your large-sized bowl and add your vinegar and oil.

4. Toss together well.

5. Serve!

Cabbage Fra Diavolo w/ Beef (Serves 8)

Ingredients:

24 ounces of Pasta Sauce

24 ounces of Ground Beef (85%)

1/2 cup of Water

1 head of Green Cabbage

Stick of Unsalted Butter

Salt

Pepper

Directions:

1. Remove and discard the outer layer of your cabbage.

2. Quarter your cabbage and shred it in your food processor.

3. Melt your butter in your large-sized pot. Add your water and cabbage. Season with your pepper and salt.

4. Cook for approximately 12 minutes. Stir occasionally.

5. While your cooking cabbage, brown your beef.

6. Add your beef to cabbage and stir in.

7. Add your pasta sauce and stir in.

8. Serve!

Cauliflower Casserole (Serves 10)

Ingredients:

12 Chicken Thighs (4 Ounces Each)

6 Thick Cut Bacon Slices

30 ounces of Chopped Cauliflower

8 ounces of Shredded Cheddar Cheese

8 ounces of Shredded Monterey Jack Cheese

6 Green Onions

1 Medium Green Pepper

8 ounces of Cream Cheese

1 Medium Onion

4 ounces of Heavy Cream

1 tablespoon of Minced Garlic

Salt

Pepper

Directions:

1. Add your chicken thighs to your casserole dish. Add your pepper and salt. Add your water to about mid thigh.

2. Cook for approximately 60 minutes at 350 degrees.

3 Cook your bacon at 450 degrees for 15 to 20 minutes.

4. Chop your cauliflower into florets. Cook your cauliflower in your microwave on the setting for your vegetables.

5. Chop your peppers and onions, Fry them in your pan.

6. Chop up your now cooked chicken into your large-sized bowl.

7. Add your other ingredients except for 2 ounces of both Monterey Jack and Cheddar.

8. Add your mixture in your greased large-sized casserole dish. Top with your remaining cheese.

9. Cover dish with your foil. Cook at 350 degrees for 25 minutes. Take off your foil and cook for an additional 5 minutes.

10. Serve!

Chicken Avocado Casserole (Serves 6)

Ingredients:

8 Cooked Boneless Chicken Thighs

8 ounces of Sour Cream

1 Medium Onion

1 Medium Pepper

8 ounces of Cheddar Cheese

4 Small Avocados

1 tablespoon of Frank's Red Hot

Salt

Pepper

Directions:

1. Preheat your oven to 350 degrees.

2. If you bought your chicken uncooked bake for approximately 90 minutes at 350 degrees.

3. Peel your avocados. Cut them in half and then slice them into thinner strips.

4. Grease your baking dish. Line the bottom of your dish with avocado slices.

5. Cut your onions and peppers into strips and fry in your pan until it is caramelized.

6. Add your chicken to your large-sized bowl and pull apart.

7. Add in your remaining ingredients.

8. Spoon your mix over your avocado slices.

9. Bake it for approximately 20 minutes.

10. Serve!

Curry Chicken w/ Riced Cauliflower (Serves 6)

Ingredients:

2 pounds of Chicken (4 Breasts)

1/2 cup of Heavy Cream

1 cup of Water

3 tablespoons of Ghee

1 packet of Curry Paste

1 head of Cauliflower

Directions:

1. Melt your ghee in your large-sized pan or pot with a lid.

2. Add your curry paste and stir well.

3. Once combined add your water and simmer for approximately 5 minutes.

4. Add your chicken. Cover your pan or pot and simmer for approximately 20 minutes.

5. While your chicken cooks, chop your cauliflower into florets and pulse it in your food processor to make it riced cauliflower.

6. Once your chicken is cooked add in your cream and cook for an additional 5 minutes.

7. Place in your bowl over your riced cauliflower.

8. Serve!

Chicken Cordon Bleu Casserole (Serves 10)

Ingredients:

3 1/3 pounds of Chicken

11 ounces of Jarlsberg Swiss Cheese

10 1/2 ounces of Ham Steak

1 cup of Cream Cheese

1 cup of Heavy Whipping Cream

Garlic Powder

Salt

Pepper

Directions:

1. Cut your chicken into 1-inch cubes. Spread them out on the bottom of your pan.

2. Season with your pepper, salt, and garlic powder.

3. Cut your ham into 1/2 inch cubes. Sprinkle them on top of your chicken.

4. Shred your Swiss cheese and spread over the top.

5. Heat your cream cheese in your microwave. Add your cream in and mix well. Pour it over your casserole.

6. Bake for approximately 40 minutes at 350 degrees.

7. Separate into 10 portions.

8. Serve!

Crockpot Buffalo Chicken (Serves 6)

Ingredients:

6 Chicken Breasts

3 tablespoons of Butter

1 bottle of Frank's Red Hot

1/2 packet of Hidden Valley Ranch

Directions:

1. Place your chicken in your crockpot.

2. Pour your hot sauce over your chicken. Sprinkle your ranch over the top of it.

3. Cover it and cook over a low heat for approximately 6 hours.

4. Shred your chicken, add your butter and cook on low uncovered for approximately 1 hour.

5. Serve!

Keto Lazy Chicken (Serves 2)

Ingredients:

2 Chicken Breasts

4 slices of Bacon

4 ounces of Cheddar Cheese

2 ounces of Jalapeno Slices

Salt

Pepper

Directions:

1. Season your chicken with your pepper and salt.

2. Cover with your cheese.

3. Add your jalapenos.

4. Cut your bacon in half and place over your chicken.

5. Place your chicken on your foil lined pan. Bake for approximately 30 to 45 minutes at 350 degrees.

6. If your chicken is cooked and your bacon is not quite done place under your broiler for a couple of minutes.

7. Serve!

Marinated Pork Chops (Serves 10)

Ingredients:

18 Pork Chops

4 tablespoons of Soy Sauce

1/2 teaspoon of Ginger

1/2 cup of Apple Cider Vinegar

1/2 cup of Splenda

1/2 teaspoon of Pepper

Directions:

1. Add all of your ingredients except your pork chops to your food processor.

2. Mix your marinade.

3. Put your pork chops in your pan that's been greased and pour your marinade on it.

4. Cook at 350 degrees for 60 minutes. Flip after approximately 30 minutes.

5. Chop your pork chops up and divide them into 10 equal portions.

6. Serve!

Cheesy Sausage Balls (Serves 12)

Ingredients:

12 ounces of Jimmy Dean's Sausage

6 ounces of Shredded Cheddar Cheese

12 cubes of Cheddar

Directions:

1. Mix your sausage and shredded cheese together.

2. Divide them up into 12 equal portions.

3. Place 1 cube of your cheese into the center of each sausage and roll them into balls.

4. Fry at 375 degrees until they get crispy.

5. Serve!

Chapter Three: Keto Diet Dinner Recipes

In this section, I will show you 30+ ketogenic dinner recipes you can cook for yourself. I'll include a few basic recipes and a few more advanced recipes. That way no matter what your level in the kitchen you'll be able to prepare a healthy low-carb high-fat keto meal to keep you on track with your diet.

Sweet Pea Coconut Hash (Serves 2)

Ingredients:

7 ounces of Stringless Sugar Snap Pea Pods

1/2 cup of Unsweetened Shredded Coconut

1/8 teaspoon of Cinnamon

1 tablespoon of Coconut Oil

4 tablespoons of Salted Butter

1 tablespoon of Rosemary Oil

Salt

Directions:

1. Melt your butter in your pan over a medium-low heat. Then add in your coconut oil.

2. Chop your pea pods into 5 slices per each pea pod.

3. Add your coconut to your pan and then mix until it is fully coated.

4. Add your rosemary oil and cinnamon. Mix until combined.

5. Cook for about 1 minute on low. This will moisten your coconut up.

6. Add your chopped pea pods and mix. Cook for approximately 5 minutes on a medium heat.

7. Add a dash of salt.

8. Serve!

Stuffed Pork Chops (Serves 4)

Ingredients:

4 Thick Cut Pork Chops

2 ounces of Cream Cheese

3 ounces of Feta Cheese

3 slices of Bacon

3 ounces of Bleu Cheese

2 ounces of Green Onion

Garlic

Salt

Pepper

Directions:

1. Cook your bacon in your skillet. Reserve your grease and put your bacon to the side.

2. Combine your feta cheese and bleu cheese in your bowl.

3. Add your green onions and bacon. Mix well.

4. Add your cream cheese and mix it until well combined.

5. Slice open your non-fatty side of your pork chop.

6. Stuff it with your cheese mixture.

7. Use a toothpick to close the opening.

8. Apply your pepper, garlic powder, and salt to the outside of your pork chops.

9. Over a high heat with your bacon grease in the pan, sear each chop for approximately 1 1/2 minutes per side.

10. Transfer your chops to your greased pan. Cook for approximately 55 minutes at 350 degrees.

11. Remove your chops and allow to rest for around 3 minutes.

12. Serve!

Roasted Tomato Shakshuka

Ingredients:

1 Large Yellow Organic Onion

1/4 cup of Organic Extra-Virgin Olive Oil

1 1/2 pounds of Organic Cherry Tomatoes

1 Red Organic Bell Pepper

4 Organic Free Range Eggs

1/2 tablespoon of Cumin Seeds

1 tablespoon of Chopped Parsley

2 Fresh Thyme Sprigs (Leaves Picked)

Sea Salt

Pinch of Cayenne

Directions:

1. Preheat your oven to 350 degrees.

2. Wash your tomatoes, cut them in 2 and lay them on your lightly oiled cookie sheet.

3. Sprinkle with your sea salt.

4. Bake for 1/2 hour or until your tomatoes are fully roasted, soft, and caramelized.

5. Heat your large-sized deep pan and dry roast your cumin seed for 1 minute.

6. Add your olive oil and your chopped onions and saute them until soft on a low flame.

7. Add your pepper cut in strips.

8. Add your herbs chopped finely.

9. Add your tomatoes, which are ideally just out of your oven, but can also be pre-made and kept in your fridge.

10. Add your salt and the cayenne pepper.

11. When your mixture is bubbling make sure there is enough water. It should be very juicy, like a sauce.

12. Carefully break your eggs around the pan, spreading them evenly.

13. Cook on the lowest flame for approximately 10 minutes, until your egg white is set but your yolk still a bit soft inside (you can vary the cook time if you prefer firmer or runnier yolks).

14. Serve!

Slow Cooker Keto Chicken Tikka Masala (Serves 5)

Ingredients:

1 1/2 pounds of Chicken Thighs (Bone-In & Skin-On)

1 pound of Chicken Thighs (Boneless & Skinless)

10-ounce can of Diced Tomatoes

3 cloves of Minced Garlic

2 tablespoons of Olive Oil

1-inch of Grated Ginger Root

2 teaspoons of Onion Powder

2 teaspoons of Smoked Paprika

5 teaspoons of Garam Masala

3 tablespoons of Tomato Paste

1 cup of Heavy Cream

1 cup of Coconut Milk (From The Carton)

1 teaspoon of Guar Gum

4 teaspoons of Kosher Salt

Chopped Fresh Cilantro

Directions:

1. De-bone your chicken on the bone-in chicken thighs. Chop all your chicken pieces into bite sized pieces. Make sure to keep the skin on for the pieces that have it. I prefer to use kitchen shears here as it makes cutting the chicken very fast and easy.

2. Add your chicken to your slow cooker and grate a 1-inch knob of ginger over the top.

3. Add all of your dry spices into your slow cooker and mix together well.

4. Add your canned diced tomatoes and tomato paste into your slow cooker, then mix again.

5. Add 1/2 cup of coconut milk and mix together thoroughly. Cook on low for approximately 6 hours or high for about 3 hours.

6. Once your slow cooker is done, add your remaining coconut milk, heavy cream, and guar gum and mix thoroughly into your chicken. It should help the curry thicken well.

7. Add over cauliflower rice or vegetables of your choice.

8. Serve!

Keto Pumpkin Carbonara (Serves 3)

Ingredients:

1 package of Shirataki Noodles

5 ounces of Pancetta

1/3 cup of Parmesan Cheese

2 Large Egg Yolks

2 tablespoons of Butter

1/2 teaspoon of Dried Sage

3 tablespoons of Pumpkin Puree

1/4 cup of Heavy Cream

Pepper

Salt

Directions:

1. Rinse off your shirataki noodles under hot water for 2 to 3 minutes. Then dry them off completely with your paper towels. Put to the side.

2. Chop your pancetta and place into your hot pan to sear on the outside.

3. Place your butter into your small-sized pot and let it brown. Once it starts to brown, mix your sage into your butter.

4. Once your sage is mixed in, add your pumpkin puree and mix together well.

5. By this point, the pancetta should be browning up nicely. Once it's crispy on the outside, remove from your pan and save the fat.

6. Add your heavy cream to your pumpkin puree sauce and mix together well until everything is combined.

7. Add your pancetta fat into your sauce and mix again until well combined. Let your sauce simmer on a medium heat.

8. Turn your pan that had you pancetta in it to high and add your shirataki noodles. Dry fry them for at least 5 minutes until a good amount of steam has come out of them.

9. Add your Parmesan cheese to your pumpkin sauce and mix together well. Turn your heat to low.

10. Continue to stir your sauce until you can scrape a spatula through the sauce and it takes a moment to come back together.

11. Add your noodles and pancetta into your sauce and toss well. Add your 2 egg yolks and mix into your sauce.

12. Add some extra Parmesan and pancetta to taste.

13. Serve!

Keto Walnut Crusted Salmon (Serves 2)

Ingredients:

2 3 ounces of Salmon Fillets

2 tablespoons of Sugar-Free Maple Syrup

1/4 teaspoon of Dill

1/2 tablespoon of Dijon Mustard

1/2 cup of Walnuts

1 tablespoons of Olive Oil

Pepper

Salt

Fresh Spinach (Optional)

Paprika (Optional)

Directions:

1. Preheat your oven to 350 degrees. Add a 1/2 cup of walnuts to your food processor.

2. Add 2 tablespoons of maple syrup and your spices.

3. Then add a tablespoon of your mustard.

4. Pulse this in your food processor until it has a paste like consistency.

5. Heat up your pan or skillet with a tablespoon of oil until it's very hot. Dry your salmon fillets thoroughly and place it skin side down in your pan. Let it sear, undisturbed for about 3 minutes.

6. While it's searing, add your walnut mixture to the top side of your salmon fillets.

7. Once they've seared, transfer them to your oven and bake for approximately 8 minutes.

8. Add some fresh spinach and paprika if you so desire.

9. Serve!

Italian Parmesan Pork Cutlets (Serves 6)

Ingredients:

6 Pork Cutlets

1/2 cup of Italian Dressing

1/2 cup of Grated Parmesan Cheese

Seasonings Of Your Choice

Directions:

1. Heat your frying pan over a medium heat.

2. Pour your Italian dressing in your bowl.

3. Pour your grated parmesan cheese in your bowl.

4. Dip your cutlets first in Italian dressing and then in your Parmesan cheese.

5. Cook your cutlets for approximately 15 minutes in your pan. Add any seasonings.

6. Serve!

Bacon & Beef Rolls (Serves 4)

Ingredients:

16 ounces of Beef

4 slices of Bacon

Montreal Steak Seasoning

Directions:

1. Preheat your oil in your deep fryer to approximately 370 degrees.

2. Cut your beef into 1x1x2-inch cubes. Should weigh 1 ounce each.

3. Take your bacon and stretch it. Cut each piece into 4 smaller-sized pieces.

4. Season your meat with your Montreal steak seasoning.

5. Wrap your beef with some bacon and skewer.

6. Cook for approximately 3 minutes in your deep fryer.

7. Serve!

Bacon Wrapped Sausages (Serves 4)

Ingredients:

5 Italian Chicken Sausages

10 slices of Bacon

Directions:

1. Preheat your deep fryer to 370 degrees.

2. Cut each of your sausages into 4 pieces.

3. Cut your bacon in half.

4. Wrap your bacon over your sausage covering up the cut end.

5. Skewer your bacon and sausage.

6. Fry it for approximately 3 to 4 minutes.

7. Serve!

Keto St. Louis Ribs

Ingredients:

2 racks of St. Louis Ribs

2 ounces of Dijon Mustard

2 tablespoons of Paprika

2 tablespoons of Splenda

1 tablespoon of Garlic Powder

1/2 tablespoon of Onion Powder

1/4 tablespoon of Cayenne Pepper

1/2 tablespoon of Ground Ginger

1/2 tablespoon of Pepper

1 tablespoon of Salt

Directions:

1. Preheat your oven to 225 degrees.

2. Remove the membrane from the back of your ribs.

3. Mix your spices together.

4. Spread your mustard over all your ribs.

5. Rub your spice mix into your meat.

6. Place your ribs on your foil-lined baking sheet.

7. Bake it uncovered for approximately 60 minutes.

8. Tent your meat with some aluminum foil. Cook for approximately 3 1/2 hours. Turn after about 2 hours.

9. Remove your foil and then broil it approximately for 5 minutes to help develop a nice crust.

10. Cover it and allow it to rest for 10 minutes.

11. Serve!

Zoodles w/ Lamb Meatballs (Serves 4)

Ingredients:

1 pound of Ground Lamb

1 pound of Zoodles (used 2 pound Zucchini)

16 ounces of Pasta Sauce

2 Shallots

1 Yolk

1 teaspoon of Cinnamon

1 teaspoon of Cumin

Red Pepper Flakes

Cayenne Pepper

Salt

Pepper

Directions:

1. Preheat your oven to 450 degrees.

2. Use your mandoline with the julienne setting and slice your zucchini into zoodles. Only slice the outer parts. Stop when you reach the seeds.

3. Mix the rest of your ingredients besides your pasta sauce. Form 16 1 ounce meatballs.

4. Cook your meatballs for approximately 12 minutes.

5. Add your sauce and zoodles to your saucepan and cook for approximately 3 to 4 minutes.

6. Serve!

Crockpot Chorizo & Chicken Soup (Serves 8)

Ingredients:

4 pounds of Boneless Skinless Chicken Thighs

1 pound of Chorizo

4 cups of Chicken Stock

1 cup of Heavy Cream

1 can of Stewed Tomatoes

2 tablespoons of Minced Garlic

2 tablespoons of Frank's Hot Sauce

2 tablespoons of Worcestershire Sauce

Sour Cream

Shaved Parmesan

Directions:

1. Brown your chorizo in your skillet.

2. Layer your ingredients in your crockpot starting with your raw chicken thighs, then chorizo and then your remaining ingredients except sour cream and shaved Parmesan.

3. Cook for approximately 3 hours on high.

4. Remove your thighs, break them apart, and place them back in your crockpot.

5. Cook for approximately 30 minutes on low heat.

6. Garnish with sour cream and shaved Parmesan.

7. Serve!

Roasted Duck (Serves 4)

Ingredients:

1 Duck

Directions:

1. Thaw your duck. Remove any excess fat. Remove any extras like the neck, heart, and liver.

2. Tie your duck legs together.

3. Cook for approximately 3 hours at 300 degrees. Turn and poke with your knife every 30 minutes. Poke through the skin but don't penetrate the meat. After 25 pokes you should see the fat oozing out of where you poked.

4. Once finished take out of your oven and quarter your roasted duck.

5. Serve!

Sous Vide Prime Rib

Ingredients:

5 Pounds of Prime Rib

Salt

Pepper

Directions:

1. Salt and pepper your meat.

2. Set your sous vide to 135 degrees.

3. Vacuum seal your prime rib.

4. Cook for approximately 10 hours.

5. Broil your finished prime rib for a few minutes.

6. Serve!

Sunflower Butter Pork Kabobs (Serves 4)

Ingredients:

1 pound of Pork Kabob Square

1 tablespoon of Soy Sauce

3 tablespoons of Sunflower Butter

1 tablespoon of Minced Garlic

2 teaspoons of Hot Sauce

1 Medium Green Pepper

1/2 teaspoon of Crushed Red Pepper

1 tablespoon of Water

Directions:

1. Place your marinade ingredients in your small-sized food processor and mix until smooth.

2. Cut your pork up into bite size squares. Place these in your non-metal bowl.

3. Mix your marinade and pork together. Allow to marinate at least 1 hour but not for more than a day.

4. Chop up your green pepper into smaller pieces.

5. Thread your pork and green pepper onto your metal skewers.

6. Broil on each side for approximately 5 minutes on high. Internal temperature should reach at least 145 degrees.

7. Serve!

Creamy Chicken w/ Spaghetti Squash (Serves 4)

Ingredients:

14 ounces of Spaghetti Squash

12 ounces of Chicken

4 ounces of Cream Cheese

5 ounces of Spinach

1 ounce of Grated Parmesan Cheese

1 tablespoon of Minced Garlic

Directions:

1. Cook your spaghetti squash.

2. Dice and then cook your 12 ounces of chicken.

3. Microwave your spinach until it is thawed and drain any excess liquid.

4. Heat up your bacon grease in your cast iron skillet

5. Add your spaghetti squash and your spinach. Saute it.

6. Add in your chicken.

7. Add your Parmesan cheese and cream cheese. Mix together well.

8. Top with your additional Parmesan cheese once cooked.

9. Serve!

BBQ Pot Roast (Serves 12)

Ingredients:

8 pounds of Beef Chuck Shoulder Roast

1 Yellow Onion

5 teaspoons of Minced Garlic

1 tablespoon of Yellow Mustard

3 tablespoons of Bacon Grease or Butter

2 tablespoons of Worcestershire Sauce

4 tablespoons of Vinegar

4 tablespoons of Splenda

1 teaspoon of Liquid Smoke

Salt

Pepper

Directions:

1. Rough chop your onion and set to the side.

2. Coat your roast with your pepper and salt.

3. Heat up your bacon grease in your pan and sear roast on each side. Approximately 1 1/2 minutes on each side.

4. Place your meat in your crockpot.

5. Fry your onions in your leftover grease. Pour this over your meat.

6. Mix together your garlic, mustard, Splenda, vinegar, liquid smoke, and Worcestershire sauce.

7. Pour this sauce over your meat.

8. Cook on low in your crockpot approximately 1 hour and 15 minutes per each pound of your roast. I cooked this one in approximately 9 hours.

9. Remove your roast from your crockpot. Separate into 12 equal-sized portions.

10. Move your liquid to your pan and reduce it by half. Add this to your meat.

11. Serve!

Bacon Wrapped Scallops (Serves 3)

Ingredients:

12 Scallops

12 Thin Bacon Slices

1 tablespoon of Oil

Salt

Pepper

12 Toothpicks

Directions:

1. Heat your skillet on a high heat with your oil.

2. Wrap each of your scallops with bacon and secure with your toothpick.

3. Season with your pepper and salt.

4. Cook for approximately 2 1/2 minutes on each side.

5. Serve!

Bacon Explosion (Serves 10)

Ingredients:

29 slices of Thick Cut Bacon

14 ounces of Steak

10 ounces of Pork Sausage

4 ounces of Shredded Cheddar Cheese

Directions:

1. Layout a 5x6-inch bacon weave in your baking dish. Bake for approximately 15 to 20 minutes at 400 degrees until nearly crisp.

2. Create your meat mixture by grinding your bacon, sausage, and steak.

3. Layout your meat in a rectangle that was the size of your first bacon weave.

4. Season your meat and then place your bacon weave on your meat.

5. Place your cheese in the center of your bacon.

6. Roll your meat into a right roll. Place in your refrigerator for a little bit.

7. Make a 7x7-inch bacon wave over your meat in a diagonal pattern.

8. Bake for approximately 50 to 60 minutes at 400 degrees. Internal temperature should reach 165 degrees.

9. Allow it to rest for approximately 10 minutes.

10. Serve!

Stuffed Peppers (Serves 2)

Ingredients:

2 Sausage Links

1 Egg

1 1/2 ounces of Parmesan Cheese

1 Small Onion

2 Green Peppers

2 ounces of Cream Cheese

2 Quail Eggs

Directions:

1. Remove your skin from your sausage and then cook your sausage into crumbles.

2. Cut off the top of your peppers and remove their seeds.

3. Chop your onions. Cook both your onions and peppers.

4. Chop your Parmesan cheese into little pieces.

5. Combine your onions, peppers, cheese, cream cheese, and sausage.

6. Stuff your peppers with your stuffing and then top it with your quail egg.

7. Cook at 400 degrees for approximately 20 minutes.

8. Serve!

Meat Pizza (Serves 4)

Ingredients:

2 Large Eggs

28 Pepperoni Slices

20 ounces of Ground Beef

1/2 cup of Shredded Cheddar Cheese

4 ounces of Mozzarella Cheese

1/2 cup of Pizza Sauce

Garlic Powder

Salt

Pepper

Directions:

1. Mix your ground beef, seasoning, and eggs together.

2. Put your ground beef into your cast iron skillet. Form it into a pizza crust.

3. Cook at 400 degrees for approximately 15 minutes.

4. Take out your crust and add your sauce, cheese, and toppings.

5. Cook until your cheese is completely melted.

6. Serve!

Sausage & Banana Pepper Fried Pizza (Serves 1)

Ingredients:

1 1/2 cups of Mozzarella Cheese

1/3 cup of Tomato Sauce

1 tablespoon of Garlic Infused Olive Oil

Grated Parmesan Cheese

Italian Seasoning

Toppings:

1/4 cup of Mozzarella Cheese

Cooked Crumbled Sausage

Chopped Yellow Onions

Chopped Banana Peppers

Directions:

1. Preheat your broiler to 500 degrees.

2. Heat a non-stick pan over a medium heat and add in your garlic oil.

3. When your oil has coated your pan, add in your mozzarella cheese.

4. Use your spatula to evenly spread your cheese and round any corners like you would a pizza.

5. Cook for approximately 3 to 5 minutes while your cheese melts and begins to get dark around the edges.

6. Once your cheese is melted add your tomato sauce gently with your spoon.

7. Cook for about 1 more minute.

8. Use your spatula and slide around the edges of your pizza and underneath to de-stick it from your pan. Don't lift it off.

9. Once your pizza is free from your pan, tip your pan and slide pizza onto a pan lined with your foil. Use a spatula to guide it.

10. Sprinkle with your Italian seasonings and grated cheese.

11. Top with 1/4 cup of mozzarella cheese, banana peppers, sausage, and onions.

12. Place in your oven approximately 2 minutes until your toppings get hot.

13. Allow it to sit for 2 minutes while your cheese hardens and begins to become like a crust.

14. Serve!

Roasted Leg of Lamb (Serves 6)

Ingredients:

3 pounds of Boneless Leg of Lamb

1 teaspoon of Thyme

2 tablespoons of Minced Garlic

1 teaspoon of Rosemary

1 tablespoon of Olive Oil

1 tablespoon of Lemon Juice

1/2 cup of Dry Red Wine

2 tablespoons of Butter

1/2 teaspoon of Pepper

Twine

Directions:

1. Preheat your oven to 450 degrees.

2. Trim the fat off the fatty side of your lamb leg.

3. Add crisscross pattern onto the fat side of your roast.

4. Mix your spices in small-sized bowl. Apply mix to each side of your roast.

5. Using twine, truss your leg of lamb so it's closed.

6. Place it on your roasting pan and cook for approximately 15 minutes at 450 degrees.

7. After about 15 minutes, turn your heat down to 325 degrees and then cook for 45 more minutes.

8. Let your meat rest for about 5 minutes.

9. Add your wine to your pan and then deglaze it.

10. Remove your twine and slice.

11. Serve!

Bourbon Glazed Ham (Serves 12)

Ingredients:

Ham:

8 to 12 Pound Bone-in Ham Shank

Glaze:

2 ounces of Bourbon

1 teaspoon of Ground Mustard

1 teaspoon of Champagne Vinegar

1 1/4 cup of Splenda

Cloves

Directions:

1. Trim your fat and then crisscross your ham.

2. Place it in your roasting pan. Add your water an inch or two high and cover. Cook for approximately 1 hour at 325 degrees.

3. Prepare your glaze combining all of your ingredients except your cloves.

4. After an hour, drain most of your water from your roasting pan.

5. Apply your glaze and place your cloves in the crisscross areas.

6. Cook for approximately 1 hour uncovered.

7. Serve!

Mac N Cheese Spaghetti Squash (Serves 6)

Ingredients:

3 Spaghetti Squash

2 ounces of Parmesan

12 ounces of Aged Cheddar

4 ounces of Cheddar

1/4 cup of Heavy Cream

1 Medium Pepper

1 Small Onion

Directions:

1. Prepare your spaghetti squash per the recipe earlier in this book.

2. Slice your onions and pepper thinly.

3. Heat your cream in your large-sized pot and add in your cheese.

4. Stir your cheese until it combines with your cream and gets smooth.

5. Add your vegetables and noodles. Mix together well.

6. Transfer your mixture to your greased casserole dish. Bake at 350 degrees for approximately 25 minutes.

7. Serve!

Reuben Casserole (Serves 4)

Ingredients:

12 ounces of Cooked Corned Beef

1 can of Sauerkraut

1 Small Onion

4 ounces of Cheddar Cheese

8 ounces of Jarlsberg

1/2 cup of Thousand Island Dressing

1/4 cup of Mayo

Pepper

Directions:

1. Slice and dice your corned beef. Add it to your large-sized bowl.

2. Use your grater with a large opening, shred your onion, and add it to your bowl.

3. Use the same grater on your Jarlsberg, add it to your bowl.

4. Drain your can of Sauerkraut. Add it to your bowl.

5. Add your cheddar cheese to your bowl.

6. Add your mayo and Thousand Island dressing to your bowl.

7. Add your fresh pepper.

8. Mix together and spread it into your 8-inch greased pan.

9. Cook for approximately 35 minutes at 350 degrees.

10. Serve!

Crockpot Corned Beef & Cabbage (Serves 10)

Ingredients:

6 pounds of Corned Beef

4 Carrots

4 cups of Water

1 Small Onion

1 Celery Bunch

1/2 teaspoon of Ground Coriander

1 Large Cabbage Head

1/2 teaspoon of Ground Mustard

1/2 teaspoon of Ground Thyme

1/2 teaspoon of Allspice

1/2 teaspoon of Ground Marjoram

1/2 teaspoon of Salt

1/2 teaspoon of Black Pepper

Directions:

1. Cut up your celery, carrots, and onions.

2. Line your crockpot with your vegetables.

3. Add your water.

4. Mix your spices all together.

5. Rub each side of your corned beef with your spices and put on top of your vegetables.

6. Cover and then cook in your crockpot on low for approximately 7 hours.

7. Discard top layer of your cabbage. Wash and then quarter.

8. Put your cabbage in your crockpot. Cook for another hour on low.

9. Serve!

Kimchi Shirataki Noodles (Serves 4)

Ingredients:

2 House Foods Tofu Shirataki Noodles

4 ounces of Sliced Pork Belly

1/2 container of Kimchi

4 stalks of Green Onions

1 tablespoon of Sesame Oil

1 tablespoon of Soy Sauce

1 tablespoon of Fish Sauce

Directions:

1. Prep your ingredients.

2. Cut your pork belly into small bite size pieces.

3. Cut your kimchi into smaller bite size pieces.

4. Wash your noodles.

5. Add your oils to your wok and heat it on high.

6. Add your pork belly and fry it for a few minutes until it's cooked.

7. Throw in your kimchi and continue to fry it.

8. Make a hole in the middle of your wok. Add your noodles. Fry until hot.

9. Transfer to your bowl and top it with your green onions.

10. Serve!

Mahi-Mahi w/ Hummus (Serves 1)

Ingredients:

1 Mahi Mahi Filet

2 tablespoons of Hummus

1 cup of Frozen Vegetables

1 teaspoon of Philadelphia Cheese

1 tablespoon of Lime

Cilantro

Fresh Coriander

Sea Salt

Ground Pepper

Directions:

1. Place your vegetables in the bottom basket and your Mahi Mahi on your top basket.

2. Add your lime, pepper, salt, and cilantro.

3. Set your steamer for approximately 30 minutes.

4. Add your cheese on your vegetables and hummus as a side dish.

5. Serve!

Coconut Shrimp & Avocado (Serves 1)

Ingredients:

1 cup of Shrimp

1/2 tablespoon of Organic Peanut Butter

1/2 Avocado

1 tablespoon of Light Coconut Milk

1 teaspoon of Shredded Coconut

Sriracha Hot Sauce

Olive Oil

Directions:

1. Set a non-stick saute pan over a medium heat. Spray with your olive oil.

2. Pour in your Sriracha, coconut milk, and peanut butter.

3. Add your shrimp and saute approximately 3 to 4 minutes until your shrimps turn pink.

4. Cut your half of an avocado into cubes and place on your plate.

5. Add your shrimps on the top of your avocado and sprinkle with your shredded coconut.

6. Serve!

Keto Baked Salmon

Ingredients:

2 pounds of Salmon Fillets

4 ounces of Sesame Oil

1/2 cup of Tamari Soy Sauce

1/2 teaspoon of Rosemary

1 teaspoon of Minced Garlic

1/2 teaspoon of Ground Ginger

1/2 teaspoon of Basil

4 ounces of Butter

1/4 teaspoon of Thyme

1 teaspoon of Oregano Leaves

1/2 teaspoon of Rosemary

1/2 cup of Chopped Fresh Mushrooms

1/4 teaspoon of Tarragon

1/2 cup of Chopped Green Onions

Directions:

1. Cut your fillet into 1/2 pound pieces. Get out a 1-quart freezer Ziploc bag.

2. Stir together your spices, sesame oil, and tamari sauce. Put your salmon in a Ziploc bag and then pour in your sauce mix.

3. Refrigerate your salmon with your skin side facing up in your marinade for 1 to 4 hours.

4. Preheat your oven to 350 degrees. Line a large-sized baking pan with your foil.

5. Pour out your fillets and marinade into your pan. Lay out your fish in a single layer.

6. Bake your fillets for approximately 10 to 15 minutes.

7. While your salmon cooks prepare your vegetables.

8. Melt your butter. Add your vegetables to it and mix to coat your vegetables.

9. Remove your salmon from your oven and pour your butter mixture over your salmon so each one is covered.

10. Bake for approximately 10 more minutes at 350 degrees.

11. Serve!

Spicy Low-Carb Kentucky Stew (Serves 14)

Ingredients:

4 pounds of Pot Roast

1 pound of Large Chicken Breast (Shredded and Boiled)

28 ounce can of Diced Tomatoes

2 teaspoon of Dried Dill Weed

2 cups of Beef Broth

7 ounces of Polish Kielbasa

1/4 teaspoon of Thyme

1 teaspoon of Basil

1/4 teaspoon of Celery Salt

1 tablespoon of Garlic Salt

2 teaspoon of Garlic Powder

1 tablespoon of Oregano

1 tablespoon of Powdered Buttermilk

1 teaspoon of Minced Garlic

1 1/2 tablespoons of Dried Parsley

1 1/2 tablespoons of Onion Powder

1 cup of Chicken Bone Broth

1/2 teaspoon of Red Pepper Flakes

1 can of Rotel Original

2 teaspoons of Frank's Red Hot Sauce

1 tablespoon of Coconut Oil

1/2 medium Chopped Onion

2 teaspoon of Pepper

Directions:

1. Add your pot roast and beef broth to your crock pot and set your temperature to low.

2. Combine your dry ingredients in your bowl and rub your pot roast on all sides with them.

3. Cook on low for approximately 4 to 8 hours.

4. Boil one large chicken breast for about 40 minutes. Shred once fully cooked. Place in your refrigerator.

5. Once your pot roast is cook split into half. 2 pounds will go to your stew. Feel free to have the other 2 pounds as a separate pot roast meal.

6. Cut your roast into cubes and place them back in your crockpot.

7. Add in the rest of your ingredients and cook on low for approximately 12 to 24 hours.

8. Flavor to taste with your hot sauce, pepper, and salt.

9. Serve!

Bacon Whiskey Caramelized Onions (Serves 1)

Ingredients:

1 Onion

1 tablespoon of Bacon Grease

3 teaspoons of Whiskey

Water

Directions:

1. Heat your pan on a medium low with your bacon grease.

2. Cut your onion in half and then cut into 1/4-inch slices.

3. Add your onions to pan once hot and cook. Use your wooden spoon to break apart onions sticking together.

4. Mix around every couple minutes for approximately 20 minutes.

5. Add a teaspoon of your whiskey followed by one teaspoon of water each time onions start getting dry and begin sticking to your pan. Mix well. Be sure to rotate using whiskey and water until all the whiskey is gone.

6. Once your onions are soft, brown, and sweet they're done. You don't want your onions to get crispy or dry. Make sure not burn.

7. Serve!

Chapter Four: Keto Diet Snacks, Drinks, & Condiment Recipes

In this section, I will show you 20+ ketogenic snacks, drinks, & condiment recipes you can cook for yourself. I'll include a few basic recipes and a few more advanced recipes. That way no matter what your level in the kitchen you'll be able to prepare a healthy low-carb high-fat keto snack, drink, or condiment to keep you on track with your diet.

Keto Pesto (Serves 1)

Ingredients:

3/4 cup of Parmesan

1/3 cup of Toasted Pine Nuts

1 1/2 cups of Basil

2 teaspoons of Tomato Paste

2/3 cup of Olive Oil

1 teaspoon of Minced Garlic

Salt

Pepper

Directions:

1. Add your fresh basil to your container.

2. Add your toasted pine nuts to the same container. Toast in your pan over a low heat if you did not get them already toasted.

3. Add the rest of your ingredients, except your oil and use your immersion blender to help blend everything all together. Add your oil slowly as blending.

4. Serve!

Guacamole (Serves 8)

Ingredients:

4 Avocados

2 Tomatoes

1/2 teaspoon of Cayenne Pepper

1 tablespoon of Minced Garlic

1 Small Onion

1 tablespoon of Lime Juice

1/2 teaspoon of Cumin

1 Jalapeno

1/2 teaspoon of Salt

Directions:

1. Peel and chop your avocados.

2. Put in your large-sized bowl and toss with your lime juice.

3 Add in your spices and mash your avocados.

4. Add your jalapenos, tomatoes, and onions. Mix together well.

5. Store at room temperature for approximately 1 hour.

6. Serve!

Keto Cheeseburger Muffins (Serves 9)

Ingredients:

Cheeseburger Muffin Buns:

2 Large Eggs

1/2 cup of Blanched Almond Flour

1/4 cup of Sour Cream

1 teaspoon of Baking Powder

1/2 cup of Flaxseed Meal

1/4 teaspoon of Pepper

1/2 teaspoon of Salt

Hamburger Filling:

16 ounces of Ground Beef

2 tablespoons of Tomato Paste

1/2 teaspoon of Garlic Powder

1/2 teaspoon of Onion Powder

Pepper

Salt

Toppings:

18 slices of Baby Dill Pickles

1/2 cup of Cheddar Cheese

2 tablespoons of Mustard

2 tablespoons of Reduced Sugar Ketchup

Directions:

1. Measure out your ground beef and place into your hot pan. Season with your salt and pepper.

2. Cook your beef until browned on the bottom, then season with your onion powder, garlic powder, and tomato paste. Mix together and turn off the heat. You should be left with "rare" (only semi-cooked) ground beef.

3. Mix together your dry ingredients for your muffins and pre-heat your oven to 350 degrees.

4. Add your wet ingredients into your muffin mixture and mix well.

5. Divide up your mixture for the muffins into silicone muffin cups. Indent your muffin using your finger or a spoon to give space for the ground beef. Then, fill each muffin with your ground beef mixture.

6. Bake for approximately 15 to 20 minutes or until your muffins are browned slightly on the outside.

7. Remove from your oven and top with some cheese, then broil for an additional 1 to 3 minutes.

8. Allow it to cool for 5 to 10 minutes, then remove from your silicone muffin cups.

9. Top with your chopped pickles, ketchup, mustard, or your favorite condiments.

10. Serve!

Personal Pan Pizza Dip (Serves 4)

Ingredients:

Personal Pan Pizza Dip:

4 ounces of Cream Cheese

1/4 cup of Parmesan Cheese

1/4 cup of Sour Cream

1/2 cup of Shredded Mozzarella Cheese

1/4 cup of Mayonnaise

1/2 cup of Shredded Mozzarella Cheese

1/2 cup of Rao's Tomato Sauce

Pepper

Salt

Pepperoni, Peppers, & Olives:

6 slices of Chopped Pepperoni

4 Pitted Sliced Black Olives

1 tablespoon of Sliced Green Pepper

1/2 teaspoon of Italian Seasoning

Pepper

Salt

Mushroom & Peppers:

2 tablespoons of Chopped Baby Bella Mushrooms

1 tablespoon of Sliced Green Pepper

1/2 teaspoon of Italian Seasoning

Salt

Pepper

Directions:

1. Pre-heat your oven to 350 degrees. Measure out your cream cheese and microwave for 20 seconds until room temperature.

2. Mix your sour cream, mayonnaise, and mozzarella cheese into your cream cheese. Season with your salt and pepper to taste.

3. Divide your mixture between 4 ramekins.

4. Spoon 2 tablespoons of Rao's Tomato Sauce over each ramekin and spread out evenly.

5. Measure out 1/2 cup of mozzarella cheese and 1/4 cup of Parmesan cheese. Sprinkle your mixture over the top of your sauce evenly, then add your toppings of choice to your personal pan pizza dips.

6. Bake for approximately 18 to 20 minutes or until your cheese is bubbling. Remove from your oven and allow it to cool for a moment.

7. Add some bread sticks or pork rinds on the side.

8. Serve!

Keto Corndog Muffins (Serves 20)

Ingredients:

1/2 cup of Blanched Almond Flour

1 Large Egg

1/2 cup of Flaxseed Meal

3 tablespoons of Swerve Sweetener

1 tablespoon of Psyllium Husk Powder

1/4 cup of Melted Butter

1/4 cup of Coconut Milk

1/4 teaspoon of Baking Powder

1/3 cup of Sour Cream

10 Smokies (or 3 Hot Dogs)

1/4 teaspoon of Salt

Spring Onion (Optional)

Directions:

1. Pre-heat your oven to 375 degrees. Mix together all of your dry ingredients in your bowl. Make sure all of your ingredients are well distributed.

2. Add your egg, sour cream, and butter and then mix well.

3. Once mixed, add your coconut milk and continue to mix.

4. Divide your batter up between 20 well-greased mini muffin slots, then cut the smokies in half and stick them in the middle.

5. Bake for approximately 12 minutes and then broil for 1 to 2 minutes until the tops are lightly browned. Feel free to use a fork or your fingers to push the pieces of the hot dog back into your muffin if they rise with your batter.

6. Allow your muffins to cool for a few minutes in your tray, then remove and allow it to cool on a wire rack.

7. Add some spring onion. You can also mix together mayonnaise, ketchup, and chili paste to make a sweet and spicy dipping sauce.

8. Serve!

Keto Tropical Smoothie (Serves 1)

Ingredients:

2 tablespoons of Golden Flaxseed Meal

1/4 cup of Sour Cream

7 Ice Cubes

1/4 cup of Sour Cream

3/4 cup of Unsweetened Coconut Milk

1 tablespoon of MCT Oil

1/2 teaspoon of Mango Extract

1/4 teaspoon of Banana Extract

1/4 teaspoon of Blueberry Extract

20 drops of Liquid Stevia

Directions:

1. Put all of your ingredients inside of your blender and wait a few minutes while your flax meal soaks up some of the moisture.

2. Blend on high speed for 1 to 2 minutes or until your consistency has thickened.

3. Serve!

Parmesan Chips (Serves 9)

Ingredients:

4 ounces of Shaved Parmesan

4 ounces of Grated Parmesan

Directions:

1. Preheat your oven to 375 degrees.

2. Layer the bottom of your well with grated cheese, followed by your shaved cheese followed by your grated cheese.

3. Cook for approximately 7 minutes until it is golden brown and crisp.

4. Allow it to cool for approximately 5 minutes.

5. Serve!

Grilled Avocado (Serves 2)

Ingredients:

1 Avocado

2 ounces of Salsa

Salt

Pepper

Directions:

1. Preheat your grill to a medium-high heat.

2. Slice your avocado in half. Remove and get rid of your pit.

3. Pepper and salt your avocado meat.

4. Put on your grill. Turn every couple minutes until your skin turns greenish and the inside has browned.

5. Add a scoop of your salsa to the center of your avocado.

6. Serve!

Grilled Garlic

Ingredients:

4 Whole Garlic Bulbs

Olive Oil

Salt

Pepper

Directions:

1. Cut tops off your garlic.

2. Soak your cloves in ice water for approximately 30 minutes.

3. Set up your grill for indirect heat. Preheat to 350 degrees.

4. Drain your garlic and put in the center of 12x12-inch square of foil. Have the cut side up.

5. Drizzle your garlic with your olive oil. Add your pepper and salt.

6. Fold the sides of your foil over to seal it.

7. Grill over your indirect heat for approximately 1 hour.

8. Serve!

Roasted Pumpkin Seeds

Ingredients:

Pumpkin Seeds

Oil

Seasoning

Directions:

1. Wash and dry your pumpkin seeds.

2. Add oil to your bowl with seeds in them. Add your seasoning. Mix well.

3. Line your pan with foil then spread your seeds out.

4. Cook at 400 degrees in your oven, stirring it at 10 minutes and then again at 20 minutes, 25 minutes, and 30 minutes.

5. After 30 minutes continue to watch until it's done.

6. Serve!

Pesto Spirals (Serves 2)

Ingredients:

1 Medium Zucchini

4 tablespoons of Pesto

5 Radishes

1/2 Large Cucumber

Directions:

1. Wash your vegetables and cut the ends off your zucchini, radishes, and cucumber.

2. Feed them into your spiralizer using the small setting.

3. Turn your vegetable to create your spirals.

4. Cut your spirals when at the desired length.

5. Add your pesto and mix well.

6. Serve!

Cheesy Pepperoni (Serves 1)

Ingredients:

7 slices of Pepperoni

1 Cheese Stick

Directions:

1. Cook your pepperoni slices in your skillet.

2. Cut your cheese stick in equal parts.

3. Place one of your cheese pieces on one of your pepperoni slices.

4. Serve!

Simple Fried Broccoli (Serves 2)

Ingredients:

2 ounces of Bleu Cheese Dressing

1 teaspoon of Frank's Red Hot

1 bunch of Broccoli

Directions:

1. Separate your broccoli into florets.

2. Deep fry them until it is crispy and golden brown.

3. Combine your hot sauce and bleu cheese as a side dipping sauce.

4. Serve!

Cheese & Chive Rollups (Serves 9)

Ingredients:

18 Slices of Thin Swiss Cheese

8-ounce package of Chive and Onion Cream Cheese

18 Slices of Ham

Directions:

1. Take out a block of your sliced ham and dry off the top slice.

2. Thinly spread out your cream cheese over your ham slices. Use 2 teaspoons per slice.

3. Scrape the last 1/2-inch of your ham clean.

4. Add a slice of cheese to the 1/2-inch non-scraped side.

5. Starting at cheese side, fold your end of ham over the end of your cheese.

6. Tightly roll your ham and cheese up.

7. Slice into small rolls.

8. Serve!

Deep Fried Jalapeno Poppers (Serves 4)

Ingredients:

<u>Inside:</u>

6 Thick Cut Bacon Slices

4 ounces of Shredded Cheddar Cheese

1 1/2 ounces of Jalapeno Slices

4 ounces of Cream Cheese

<u>Batter:</u>

2 Eggs

2 tablespoons of Parmesan Cheese

1 tablespoon of Water

4 tablespoons of Almond Flour

Directions:

1. Cook your bacon and crumble it.

2. Chop your jalapeno slices.

3. Combine your bacon, cheddar cheese, jalapeno slices, and cream cheese.

4. Form into 20 equal sized balls. Place in your refrigerator.

5. Make your batter by whisking your eggs, adding in your Parmesan cheese and almond flour.

6. Coat your balls. Refrigerate again.

7. Fry your balls until they turn golden brown.

8. Serve!

Simple Fried Zucchini

Ingredients:

Zucchini

Salt

Directions:

1. Heat your fryer to 375 degrees.

2 Wash your zucchini then cut off their ends.

3. Slice your zucchini thinly into chips or fries. The thinner you make them the better.

4. Fry until they turn golden brown. Turn occasionally when frying.

5. Serve!

Open Faced Quail Egg Sandwich (Serves 3)

Ingredients:

10 Quail Eggs

2 1/2 slices of Cheddar Cheese

5 slices of Bacon

Salt

Pepper

Standard Almond Bun:

2 Eggs

1 1/2 teaspoons of Baking Powder

1 1/2 teaspoons of Splenda

5 tablespoons of Unsalted Water

3/4 cup of Almond Flour

Directions:

1. Mix your almond bun ingredients together. Divide into 10 separate portions on a pie pan.

2. Bake at 350 degrees for approximately 8 to 12 minutes.

3. Cook your bacon.

4. Fry your 10 quail eggs. Top them with your pepper and salt.

5. Top each of your almond buns with 1/4 slice of cheese, 1/2 slice of bacon, and one quail egg.

6. Serve!

Goat Cheese & Zucchini Wraps (Serves 6)

Ingredients:

1 Zucchini

6 ounces of Soft Goat Cheese

1 teaspoon of Dried Mint

1 teaspoon of Dried Dill

Oil

Salt

Pepper

Toothpicks

Directions:

1. Wash your zucchini and cut off the ends.

2. Using your mandoline, slice your zucchini into 1/8-inch slices.

3. Brush your slices with your oil and add pepper and salt.

4. Grill for approximately 5 minutes turning over at the halfway point.

5. Combine your mint, dill, and goat cheese.

6. Divide your mixture into 6 servings.

7. Roll your goat cheese into cylinder shape between fingers and spread on zucchini.

8. Roll up your zucchini and stick a toothpick through it.

9. Serve!

Deviled Egg Chicks (Serves 10)

Ingredients:

10 Eggs

4 tablespoons of Mayo

1 tablespoon of Dijon Mustard

Olive Slivers

Carrot Slivers

Dash of Hot Sauce

Directions:

1. Place your eggs in your pan and cover with water.

2. Boil your eggs for 15 minutes.

3. Shock your eggs with cold water and peel them.

4. Slice your eggs in half and separate out your egg yolks.

5. In your mixing bowl, combine your mayo, egg yolks, hot sauce, and mustard.

6. Whisk until smooth.

7. Cut the bottom half of your egg halves and middle out the rest of them.

8. Pipe in your yolk mix on the bottoms, adding more to the front.

9. Top with the rest of your egg and add your carrot and two olive slices.

10. Serve!

Bacon Deviled Eggs (Serves 20)

Ingredients:

10 Large Eggs

1 tablespoons of Sugar-Free Pickle Relish

5 tablespoons of Mayo

4 slices of Thick Cut Bacon

Paprika

Directions:

1. Hard boil your eggs.

2. Cover your eggs with cold water an inch above them.

3. Apply high heat and once your water boils. Boil for approximately 15 minutes.

4. Carefully remove your water and cover your eggs with cold water.

5. Crack your eggs all around and roll between hands to peel.

6. Dry your peeled eggs.

7. Cut your eggs lengthwise in half. Separate your yolks from your egg whites.

8. In your large-sized mixing bowl, crumble your yolks using a fork.

9. Add your mayo until your mixture gets a batter consistency.

10. Add your pickle relish and mix well.

11. Add the cooled, crumbled up bacon.

12. Using your fork, fill your egg halves with your yolk mixture.

13. Sprinkle your deviled eggs with your paprika.

14. Serve!

Mashed Cauliflower (Serves 6)

Ingredients:

5 slices of Bacon

1 head of Cauliflower

2 ounces of Cream Cheese

2 1/2 ounces of Cheddar Cheese

2 1/2 ounces of Monterey Jack Cheese

Salt

Pepper

Directions:

1. Cook your bacon and crumble.

2. Wash, remove your leaves and chop your cauliflower.

3. Bring your water to boil, add your cauliflower and boil for approximately 9 minutes.

4. Cube your cheeses while your cauliflower boils.

5. Drain your cauliflower.

6. Mash your cauliflower, add your cream cheese and then mash it again.

7. Season with your pepper and salt.

8. Stir in your bacon and cheese. You can stop there or you can also place in your baking dish and bake for approximately 10 minutes at 350 degrees.

9. Serve!

Garlic Asparagus (Serves 4)

Ingredients:

1 bunch of Asparagus

1 tablespoon of Minced Garlic

2 tablespoons of Butter

Directions:

1. Wash your asparagus then separate your stalks.

2. Boil your water and cook your asparagus for 2 to 3 minutes.

3. Drain your asparagus and then cool them down in your cold water.

4. Heat your butter and your garlic in your skillet.

5. Fry your asparagus until browning and crisp.

6. Serve!

Peppery Cheese Biscuits (Serves 37)

Ingredients:

2 Large Eggs

6 ounces of Shredded Colby Jack Cheese

2 1/2 cups of Almond Flour

5 tablespoons of Butter

8 ounces of Cream Cheese

1 teaspoon of Baking Soda

3/4 teaspoon of Xanthan Gum

3 teaspoons of Freshly Cracked Black Pepper

1 teaspoon of Sea Salt

Directions:

1. Preheat your oven to 325 degrees. Line your cookie sheet with your parchment paper.

2. Put 1 cup of almond flour and shredded cheese in your food processor. Process until it is finely grained. Put to the side.

3. In your glass mixing bowl, place your cream cheese and butter. Microwave 30 seconds and remove. Whisk it until it is glossy and smooth.

4. Whisk in your eggs until your mixture is smooth. Mix in your baking soda, pepper, salt, and xanthan gum.

5. Add your almond flour cheese mix to egg mixture. Add your remaining almond flour and fold in until mixed together well and a dough begins forming.

6. Drop your mixture by the tablespoon onto your cookie sheet. Space each an inch apart. Roll your dough a bit to smooth it out so it makes a prettier biscuit.

7. Bake for approximately 20 to 25 minutes. Should be golden brown on top. Remove and allow it to cool down for approximately 10 minutes. Makes about 37 biscuits.

8. Serve!

Coffee Smoothie (Serves 2)

Ingredients:

6 ounces of Cold Coffee

4 ounces of Unsweetened Milk

2 tablespoons of Unsweetened Cocoa

4 ounces of Heavy Cream

1 ounce of Torani Sugar-Free Chocolate Syrup

1 ounce of Torani Sugar-Free Caramel Syrup

16 ounces of Ice

Directions:

1. Add your liquids to your blender, then add your powder and finally your ice.

2. Use the smoothie setting on your Vitamix with your tamper attachment to push your mix towards your blades.

3. Serve!

Avocado Shake (Serves 1)

Ingredients:

1 Avocado

3 ounces of Unsweetened Almond Milk

3 ounces of Heavy Whipping Cream

6 drops of EZ-Sweetz

6 Ice Cubes

Directions:

1. Add almond milk, EZ-Sweetz, and heavy whipping cream to your Vitamix.

2. Cut your avocado in half and remove the seed. Remove the flesh from your skin and add to your mixer.

3. Add in your 6 ice cubes.

4. Blend on your smoothie setting. For regular blender keep blending until your mixture has a yogurt consistency.

5. Serve!

Raspberry Lemonade Poptail (Serves 2)

Ingredients:

60 milliliters of Heavy Cream

20 milliliters of Vodka

25 milliliters of Torani Sugar-Free Raspberry Syrup

10 milliliters of Lemon Juice

5 milliliters of Vanilla

Directions:

1. Freeze your Zoku device 24 hours until fully frozen.

2. Each popsicle uses 60 milliliters of your total mix.

3. Mix your ingredients and then place in your freezer.

4. Bring out your Zoku device and place your popsicle stick into it.

5. Add your liquid and wait for approximately 16 minutes. May take a little longer to freeze due to the alcohol in it.

6. Once completely frozen, screw on your extractor and release from the mold.

7. Snap your drip shield on.

8. Serve!

Whipped Eggnog (Serves 4)

Ingredients:

3/4 cup of Heavy Cream

1/4 cup of Bourbon

2 Egg Yolks

18 drops of EZ-Sweetz

Ground Nutmeg

Directions:

1. Mix your ingredients in your bowl.

2. I use an iSi Mini Whip to make my whip cream. Charge up the charger and add it to your canister.

3. Pressurize it with your nitrogen.

4. Shake it 3 to 4 times.

5. Pour into your bowl.

6. Dust with nutmeg.

7. Serve!

Alcohol-Infused Whipped Cream (Serves 10)

Ingredients:

200 milliliters of Heavy Cream

50 milliliters of Vanilla Vodka

1/4 teaspoon of Vanilla

1/4 teaspoon of EZ-Sweetz

Directions:

1. Combine all of your ingredients and place in your iSi Mini Easy Whip Container.

2. Charge it with your nitrogen cartridge.

3. Shake 3 to 4 times, if it comes out a little runny just shake some more.

4. Pour into your bowl or on top of drink or dessert.

5. Serve!

Keto Margaritas

Ingredients:

1 Lime

1 1/2 ounces of Tequila

4 drops of Sucralose

Directions:

1. Cut your lime in half and squeeze it into your container.

2. Fill an old fashion glass with your regular ice or crushed ice.

3. Measure 1 1/2 ounces of lime juice into your glass.

4. Measure 1 1/2 ounces of tequila into your glass.

5. Add 4 drops of sucralose.

6. Mix and then garnish with a lime slice.

7. Serve!

Simple Cheese Dip (Serves 12)

Ingredients:

2 pounds of Extra Sharp Cheddar

1 Small Onion

16 ounces of Mayo

8 dashes of Frank's Red Hot

3 tablespoons of Lemon Juice

1 tablespoon of Worcestershire Sauce

Directions:

1. Shred your cheddar cheese and place it in your large-sized mixing bowl.

2. Shred your onions and add it to your bowl.

3. Add in all your other ingredients.

4. Mix together well.

5. Serve!

Chapter Five: Keto Diet Dessert Recipes

In this section, I will show you 20+ ketogenic dessert recipes you can cook for yourself. I'll include a few basic recipes and a few more advanced recipes. That way no matter what your level in the kitchen you'll be able to prepare a healthy low-carb high-fat keto dessert to keep you on track with your diet.

Quest Cookies (Serves 1)

Ingredients:

1 Quest Bar

Directions:

1. Preheat your oven to 450 degrees.

2. Microwave bar for 10 seconds.

3. Break into 8 evenly sized parts and roll up into balls.

4. Put on your baking sheet and cook for approximately 3 minutes.

5. Serve!

Pumpkin Pie Fat Bombs (Serves 15)

Ingredients:

2 ounces of Coconut Butter

1/4 cup of Erythritol

1/2 cup of Pumpkin Puree

2 teaspoons of Pumpkin Pie Spice

1/2 cup of Chopped Pecans

1/2 cup of Coconut Oil

Directions:

1. Melt your coconut oil if not already a liquid. Melt your coconut butter so it's soft and easy to work with.

2. Combine your coconut butter, coconut oil, and pumpkin puree in your mixing bowl. Stir well until all combined together.

3. Add your erythritol.

4. Add your pumpkin pie spice.

5. Add your batter mixture to candy molds, ice cube trays, or containers.

6. Toast some of your chopped pecans over a medium heat in your dry pan until fragrant and slightly browned.

7. Top each of your fat bombs with pecan pieces and press them in gently so they stick.

8. Refrigerate until they all set.

9. Serve!

Coconut Orange Creamsicle Fat Bombs (Serves 10)

Ingredients:

1/2 cup of Coconut Oil

4 ounce of Cream Cheese

1/2 cup of Heavy Whipping Cream

10 drops of Liquid Stevia

1 teaspoon of Orange Vanilla Mio

Directions:

1. Measure out your coconut oil, heavy cream, and cream cheese.

2. Use an immersion blender to blend together all of your ingredients. If you're having a hard time blending your ingredients, you can microwave them for 30 seconds to 1 minute to soften them up.

3. Add Orange Vanilla Mio and liquid stevia into your mixture, and mix together with a spoon.

4. Spread your mixture into a silicone tray and freeze for 2 to 3 hours.

5. Once hardened, remove from your silicone tray and store in your freezer.

6. Serve!

Savory Pizza Fat Bombs (Serves 6)

Ingredients:

14 slices of Pepperoni

4 ounces of Cream Cheese

8 Pitted Black Olives

2 tablespoons of Sun Dried Tomato Pesto

2 tablespoons of Chopped Fresh Basil

Pepper

Salt

Directions:

1. Dice your pepperoni and olives into small pieces.

2. Mix together your basil, tomato pesto, and cream cheese.

3. Add your olives and pepperoni into your cream cheese and mix again.

4. Form into balls, then garnish with your pepperoni, basil, and olive.

5. Serve!

No Bake Chocolate Peanut Butter Fat Bombs (Serves 8)

Ingredients:

1/2 cup of Coconut Oil

6 tablespoons of Shelled Hemp Seeds

1/4 cup of Cocoa Powder

1/4 cup of Unsweetened Shredded Coconut

4 tablespoons of PB Fit Powder

1 teaspoon of Vanilla Extract

2 tablespoons of Heavy Cream

28 drops of Liquid Stevia

Directions:

1. Mix together all of your dry ingredients with your coconut oil. It may take a bit of work, but it will eventually turn into a paste.

2. Add your heavy cream, vanilla, and liquid stevia. Mix again until everything is combined and slightly creamy.

3. Measure out your unsweetened shredded coconut onto a plate.

4. Roll balls out using your hand and then roll in your unsweetened shredded coconut. Lay onto a baking tray covered in your parchment paper. Set in your freezer for about 20 minutes.

5. Serve!

Raspberry Lemon Popsicles (Serves 6)

Ingredients:

3 1/2 ounces of Raspberries

1/4 cup of Coconut Oil

1/4 cup of Heavy Cream

1 cup of Coconut Milk (From The Carton)

1/2 teaspoon of Guar Gum

1/4 cup of Sour Cream

20 drops of Liquid Stevia

Juice of 1/2 Lemon

Directions:

1. Add all of your ingredients into a container and use an immersion blender to blend your mixture together.

2. Continue blending until your raspberries are completely mixed in with the rest of your ingredients.

3. Strain your mixture, making sure to discard all raspberry seeds.

4. Pour the mixture into your molds. I use this mold for my popsicles. Set the popsicles in your freezer for a minimum of 2 hours.

5. Run your mold under hot water to dislodge your popsicles.

6. Serve!

White Chocolate Butter Pecan Fat Bombs (Serves 4)

Ingredients:

2 ounces of Cocoa Butter

2 tablespoons of Butter

2 tablespoons of Coconut Oil

1/2 cup of Chopped Pecans

2 tablespoons of Powdered Erythritol

1/4 teaspoon of Vanilla Extract

Pinch of Salt

Pinch of Stevia

Directions:

1. Melt your butter, coconut butter, and coconut oil together in your pan until it is melted. Turn off the heat.

2. Add your powdered erythritol to your butter mixture and stir well.

3. Add a pinch of salt, Stevia, and vanilla extract.

4. Add some of your chopped pecans to your silicone cupcake molds or candy molds.

5. Pour your white chocolate mix into your molds evenly and place them in your freezer.

6. Freeze for approximately 30 minutes.

7. Serve!

Mexican Chocolate Pudding (Serves 2)

Ingredients:

1 tablespoon of Coconut Milk

2 1/2 tablespoons of Raw Cocoa Powder

1 Avocado

1 teaspoon of Ceylon Cinnamon

1 tablespoon of Coconut Milk

1/16 teaspoon of Ground Cayenne Pepper

1/2 teaspoon of Pure Vanilla Extract

1 tablespoon of Sweetener

Pinch of Pink Himalayan Sea Salt

Pinch of Stevia

Directions:

1. Cut and pit your avocado. Blend in your food processor until smooth.

2. Add your coconut milk, vanilla extract, and cocoa powder. Blend it until it is smooth.

3. Add your cinnamon, sweetener, ground cayenne pepper, and Stevia.

4. Blend until smooth. Get rid of all the chunks.

5. Sprinkle with your sea salt.

6. Serve!

Almond Joy Fat Bombs (Serves 15)

Ingredients:

15 Almonds

1/4 cup of Shredded Coconut

1 tablespoon of Coconut Oil

1/2 of Low-Carb Chocolate Bar

1 tablespoon of Erythritol

Heart Shaped Candy Mold

Directions:

1. Melt your chocolate bar. Pour half a teaspoon of your melted chocolate bar into your candy mold and add an almond to each.

2. Freeze and start working on the next step.

3. Combine your shredded coconut and your coconut oil. Then add your erythritol and combine together.

4. Add a teaspoon of coconut mixture to candy molds and gently press to create a flat layer on top.

5. Freeze for another 5 minutes so your coconut oil solidifies.

6. Finish your candies off using the rest of your chocolate mixture and then smooth out the top of your candy mold.

7. Freeze for at least 1 hour.

8. Pop out your candies.

9. Serve!

Blueberry Lemon Shortbread Cookies (Serves 9)

Ingredients:

Cookies:

1 Egg

1/4 cup of Softened Butter

1/2 cup of Sukrin Sweetener

1 tablespoon of Lemon Juice

1 Egg Yolk

3/4 cup of Sifted Almond Flour

1 teaspoon of Vanilla Extract

1/2 teaspoon of Xanthan Gum

1/2 teaspoon of Baking Powder

1 tablespoon of Coconut Flour

1/2 teaspoon of Salt

Blueberry Glaze:

1/4 cup of Blueberries

2 tablespoons of Sukrin Melis

1/4 cup of Coconut Oil

Directions:

1. Preheat your oven to 350 degrees.

2. Beat together your butter and Sukrin until it is creamy.

3. Add in your egg yolk and egg along with your vanilla and lemon juice. Mix it well.

4. In a different bowl, sift your almond flour and combine with the rest of your dry ingredients excluding your xanthan gum.

5. Slowly pour your dry ingredients into wet ingredients, beating your mixture the entire time.

6. When all combined add your xanthan gum and mix it well.

7. Line your baking sheet using your parchment paper and measure out evenly sized cookie dough balls. Flatten each one and ensure each one cooks evenly.

8. Bake for approximately 8 to 10 minutes.

9. Allow it to cool completely.

10. Make your glaze. Combine all of your ingredients in your immersion blender or Nutribullet.

11. Allow glaze to sit and thicken up. Put a teaspoon of glaze over each of your cookies.

12. Refrigerate your glazed cookies for an hour.

13. Serve!

Cinnamon Coconut Peanut Butter Cookies (Serves 15)

Ingredients:

1 Egg

1/4 cup of Butter

1 cup of Peanut Butter

2 tablespoons of Shredded Coconut

1/2 cup of Erythritol

1 tablespoon of Cinnamon

1/2 teaspoon of Vanilla Extract

Pinch of Salt

Directions:

1. Preheat your oven to 350 degrees. Beat together your butter, peanut butter, erythritol, and egg.

2. Add in your cinnamon, shredded coconut, salt and fold it all in together.

3. Roll into balls about 1 1/2-inches in diameter. Lay out on your baking sheet lined with parchment paper.

4. Sprinkle with your shredded coconut.

5. Bake for approximately 15 minutes. Edges should become golden colored.

6. Allow it to cool.

7. Serve!

Keto Ice Cream (Serves 4)

Ingredients:

8 Strawberries

1/2 cup of Heavy Cream

3 ounces of Cream Cheese

16 drops of EZ-Sweetz

1/4 teaspoon of Vanilla Extract

1 tablespoon of Lemon Juice

3/4 cup of Ice

Directions:

1. Place your ingredients in your Vitamix.

2. Using the variable speed setting, start on 1 until your solids are pulverized then rotate to 10 slowly while you use your tamper to push your ingredients into the blades. Blend together for 30 to 60 seconds until mounds begin to form.

3. Serve!

Keto Popsicles (Serves 2)

Ingredients:

4 tablespoons of Heavy Cream

2 1/3 tablespoons of Sugar-Free Coconut Milk

4 teaspoons of Sugar-Free Flavored Syrup

Directions:

1. Freeze your Zoku device for approximately 1 day or until completely frozen.

2. Each popsicle will use 4 tablespoons of your total mix. Mix ingredients and put in your freezer.

3. Bring out your Zoku and place a popsicle stick in it.

4. Add your liquid and wait for approximately 9 minutes.

5. Once completely frozen, screw in your extractor and release mold.

6. Snap on your drip shield.

7. Serve!

Keto Chocolate Cheesecake (Serves 8)

Ingredients:

Chocolate Crust:

1 cup of Almond Flour

4 tablespoons of Butter

1 tablespoon of Cocoa Powder

1/2 teaspoon of Cinnamon

1/16 teaspoon of Stevia

Pinch of Salt

Cheesecake Filling:

16 ounces of Softened Cream Cheese

2 Eggs

1/2 cup of Sour Cream

3/4 cup of Erythritol

1 teaspoon of Vanilla Extract

1 tablespoon of Cocoa Powder

3 ounces of Unsweetened Baker's Chocolate

Pinch of Salt

Directions:

1. Preheat your oven to 350 degrees.

2. Melt your butter and combine with your cinnamon, almond flour, Stevia, and cocoa powder. Mix together well.

3. Press this crust dough mixture into 9-inch springform pan and bake for approximately 15 minutes until your crust becomes solid and gets darker.

4. Begin making your cream cheese filling while your crust bakes. Beat your erythritol and cream cheese with an electric hand mixer until it is smooth.

5. Add in your vanilla extract, sour cream, eggs, and salt. Beat with your mixer until it gets creamy.

6. Melt your baker's chocolate in a small-sized pan over a low heat. Stir it constantly.

7. Pour your chocolate and cocoa powder into your cream cheese mixture. Stir with your spatula to combine your two mixtures.

8. Pour your cheesecake batter into your pan on top of the crust.

9. Bake for approximately 50 to 60 minutes until your cheesecake sets.

10. Allow it to cool. I like to refrigerate it overnight.

11. Run your knife around the edges of your pan to loosen cake.

12. Serve!

Mini Cheesecakes (Serves 8)

Ingredients:

Cheesecake:

1 Egg

1/2 teaspoon of Lemon Juice

8 ounces of Cream Cheese

1/2 teaspoon of Vanilla Extract

1/4 cup of Erythritol

Pinch of Salt

Crust:

1/2 cup of Almond Meal

2 tablespoons of Butter

Directions:

1. Preheat your oven to 350 degrees.

2. To make your crust, melt your butter until it is liquid and then mix with your almond meal.

3. Take a teaspoon of your dough at a time and press into the bottom of your muffin tin. You can line your pan with cupcake liners to make removal easy.

4. Bake your crusts for approximately 5 minutes at 350 degrees. Should be crispy and slightly brown.

5. Beat your cream cheese with your electric hand mixer until it is creamy. Add your lemon, vanilla extract, erythritol, and egg. Beat until well combined.

6. Fill all the crust bottomed muffin tin cups. Do so evenly and nearly to the top.

7. Bake for approximately 15 minutes at 350 degrees. Cheesecakes should be a little jiggly.

8. Allow it to cool. I let them cool overnight.

9. Slide a knife around your outer edges of each cup to loosen.

10. Serve!

Chocolate Cherry Cheesecake

Ingredients:

8 ounces of Softened Cream Cheese

2 ounces of Heavy Cream

1 teaspoon of Stevia Glycerite

1 tablespoon of Dutch Process Cocoa Powder

1 tablespoon of Da Vince Sugar-Free Cherry Flavored Syrup

5 drops of EZ-Sweet Liquid

Directions:

1. Mix all your ingredients together except EZ-Sweet and then whip it into a pudding-like consistency.

2. Add your EZ-Sweet a drop at a time to your mixture until it is sweet. Spoon your mixture into small-sized serving cups and then refrigerate until it sets.

3. Serve!

Chocolate Peanut Butter Truffles

Ingredients:

4 tablespoons of Melted Butter

1 1/2 cups of Powdered Erythritol

1 cup of Peanut Butter

6 ounces of Sugar-Free Chocolate

Directions:

1. Melt your butter.

2. Mix your peanut butter, powdered erythritol, and melted butter together.

3. Scoop out 2 tablespoons of your mixture and roll out into small balls. Lay on your baking sheet lined with parchment paper. Chill in your refrigerator for approximately 30 minutes.

4. Melt your chocolate in your small-sized bowl for 10 to 20 seconds in your microwave. Stir it well.

5. Place one of your truffles in your bowl at a time and rotate it with a spoon so that chocolate covers every side. Take out and allow excess chocolate to fall off.

6. Place back on your baking sheet lined with parchment paper and place in refrigerator for another hour to chill.

7. Serve!

Flourless Chocolate Cake (Serves 8)

Ingredients:

3 Eggs

1 teaspoon of Vanilla Extract

4 ounces of Unsweetened Baker's Chocolate

1/2 cup of Butter

1/2 cup of Cocoa Powder

1 cup of Swerve Erythritol (separated into 1/2 cup, 1/4 cup, 1/4 cup)

1/2 teaspoon of Salt

Directions:

1. Preheat your oven to 300 degrees. Set up your double boiler to melt your butter and baker's chocolate together. If no boiler use your pan over a low heat.

2. Once they are both melted, combine them both together. Add in 1/2 cup of erythritol and stir well over a low flame until it is dissolved.

3. Separate 3 eggs and beat your eggs whites until they get foamy. Add 1/4 cup of erythritol slowly while beating your egg whites. Should form stiff peaks and turn glossy.

4. Clean beaters and beat your 3 egg yolks. Slowly add in last 1/4 cup of erythritol. Yolks should turn pale yellow and double in volume.

5. Add in your chocolate mixture to egg yolks. Stir well.

6. Add in your cocoa powder. Stir well. Add your salt and vanilla.

7. Add a third of your egg whites and fold in gently. Repeat process until all your eggs whites have been added and folded in.

8. Spray your springform pan with some cooking oil. Pour in your chocolate batter. Bake for approximately 35 minutes.

9. Dust with some powdered erythritol.

10. Serve!

Sugar-Free Panna Cotta (Serves 4)

Ingredients:

1 cup of Unsweetened Almond Milk

1/3 cup of Erythritol

1 cup of Heavy Cream

1 tablespoon of Fresh Lemon Juice

1 sachet of Unflavored Gelatin

1/2 cup of Sugar-Free Raspberry Jam

1 teaspoon of Vanilla Extract

Raspberries

Directions:

1. In your saucepan, combine your almond milk and heavy cream over a low flame.

2. Add your gelatin and erythritol. Allow it to dissolve in your warm cream. Don't allow it to boil.

3. Use your whisk to stir it together well.

4. Turn off the heat and add your lemon juice and vanilla extract.

5. Grease 4 cups or ramekins. Spray with your oil and pour your batter into each one evenly.

6. Cover your cup or ramekin with plastic wrap and place in your refrigerator for a minimum of 2 hours.

7. Take out and run a knife around the edges. Flip over onto a plate.

8. Top with your raspberry jam and fresh raspberries.

9. Serve!

Pumpkin Maple Flaxseed Muffins (Serves 10)

Ingredients:

1 Egg

1/2 tablespoon of Baking Powder

1/3 cup of Erythritol

1 tablespoon of Pumpkin Pie Spice

1/2 teaspoon of Apple Cider Vinegar

1 1/4 cups of Ground Flaxseeds

1 cup of Pure Pumpkin Puree

1 tablespoon of Cinnamon

1/4 cup of Walden Farm's Maple Syrup

1/2 teaspoon of Vanilla Extract

2 tablespoons of Coconut Oil

1/2 teaspoon of Salt

Directions:

1. Add some cupcake liners to your muffin tin. Preheat your oven to 350 degrees.

2. Grind your flaxseeds for 1 second in your Nutribullet.

3. Combine your dry ingredients and stir well to disperse evenly.

4. Add your pumpkin puree. Mix well.

5. Add your vanilla extract, maple syrup, and pumpkin spice.

6. Add your coconut oil, apple cider vinegar mix, and egg. Mix well.

7. Add a large tablespoon of mixture to each muffin liner and top with your pumpkin seeds. Allow for some room for your muffins to rise.

8. Bake for approximately 20 minutes. Tops should brown slightly.

9. Allow it to cool. Add any toppings or butter to muffins.

10. Serve!

Keto Truffles (Serves 12)

Ingredients:

2 tablespoons of Honey

5 1/4 ounces of Organic Dark Chocolate

2 tablespoons of Grass Fed Butter

1/2 teaspoon of Pure Vanilla Extract

1/2 cup of Organic Heavy Cream

1/2 teaspoon of Cinnamon

2 tablespoons of Raw Cocoa Powder

Pinch of Sea Salt

Directions:

1. Heat your cream over the low flame. Don't allow it to boil.

2. Chop your chocolate into small pieces.

3. When simmering add in your chocolate and stir until it is combined with cream. Add in your butter and stir in until it is melted completely.

4. Turn off your heat and add your cinnamon, vanilla, honey, and salt. Mix well to combine.

5. Place in your refrigerator for approximately 1 hour. Stir every 20 minutes.

6. Once cooled and hardened, scoop some of your mixture out and roll into small balls about 1 1/2-inches in diameter.

7. Place each truffle ball on your baking sheet lined with parchment paper and refrigerate for approximately 30 minutes.

8. Roll in hands to smooth balls out. Place your cocoa powder in your bowl and add your truffles. Shake and roll them in your cocoa powder to coat evenly.

9. Serve!

Keto Apple Pie (Serves 8)

Ingredients:

Crust:

4 Eggs

1 1/2 cups of Coconut Flour

1 cup of Grass Fed Butter

1/2 teaspoon of Salt

Filling:

1/4 cup of Honey

1 tablespoon of Cinnamon

6 Macintosh Apples

2 tablespoons of Grass Fed Butter

1 teaspoon of Vanilla Extract

Directions:

1. Preheat your oven to 425 degrees.

2. Melt 1 cup of grass fed butter and combine with your eggs and whisk it together.

3. Add your salt and coconut flour.

4. Divide your mixture in half and roll one of your halves into a ball and press and flatten it to your greased 9-inch pie pan.

5. With your other 1/2 of dough, roll and flatten into 1/4-inch of thickness. Place to the side.

6. Peel and slice your apples into desired size pieces.

7. Toss your apple pieces, vanilla extract, honey, and cinnamon into your bowl. Make sure apples are all evenly coated in your mixture.

8. Pour your apples into your crust-lined pan. Place your butter on top to allow it to brown and moisten your filling. Cover piece with your rolled out dough that you put to the side. Seal all the edges by pinching them. Slice a few slits on top of your dough so some steam can come out in the oven when cooking.

9. Separate an egg. Whisk the white part. Use a kitchen brush to brush some of your egg on the entire top crust.

10. Place in your oven and bake for approximately 15 minutes at 425 degrees. Lower to 350 degrees and continue baking for another 40 minutes.

11. Allow it to cool slightly until it is warm.

12. Serve!

Nutella Sundae (Serves 2)

Ingredients:

4 scoops of Low-Carb Ice Cream

2 tablespoons of Homemade Nutella

2 Strawberries

Sprinkles

Whipped Cream

Directions:

1. Mix it all together.

2. Place in your bowl.

3. Add your toppings.

4. Serve!

Conclusion

Thanks for reading my book. I hope this keto diet cookbook has provided you with a nice variety of recipes for every meal to get you started off on the right track. I hope you enjoy all the delicious recipes I've included.

Good luck. I wish you nothing but the best!

Made in the USA
San Bernardino, CA
06 June 2017